Women's Health

The Daily Fix

Women'sHealth.

The Daily Fix

YOUR GUIDE TO HEALTHY HABITS FOR GOOD NUTRITION

ALEXA L. FISHBACK, MS, RD

RODALE

© 2008 by Alexa Fishback, MS, RD

All rights reserved. No part of this publication may be reproduced or transmitted in any form or by any means, electronic or mechanical, including photocopying, recording, or any other information storage and retrieval system, without the written permission of the publisher.

Women's Health is a registered trademark of Rodale Inc.

Printed in the United States of America

Rodale Inc. makes every effort to use acid-free ♾, recycled paper ♻.

Library of Congress Cataloging-in-Publication Data
Fishback, Alexa L.
 The daily fix / Alexa L. Fishback.
  p.   cm.
 Includes bibliographical references and index.
 ISBN-13 978-1-59486-847-4 hardcover
 ISBN-10 1-59486-847-6 hardcover
 1. Women white collar workers—Nutrition.   2. Women white collar workers—Health and hygiene.   I. Title.
 RA778.F49 2008
 613`.04244—dc22   2008037990

2 4 6 8 10 9 7 5 3 1   hardcover

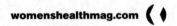

womenshealthmag.com

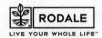

We inspire and enable people to improve their lives and the world around them

For more of our products visit **rodalestore.com** or call 800-848-4735

Contents

Part 4: Evening

Part 5: Lifestyle

Introduction

As a working woman, I have a unique set of concerns about my health, nutrition, and body that seem strangely under-represented in the abundance of wellness and diet literature that lines the shelves of our bookstores. As a nutritionist, friend, and sister, I realize that many women share a similar set of grievances and are eager for a resource that speaks directly to their needs. We want intelligent strategies to combat the health issues we face every day. For instance, how do we avoid gaining a few pounds after starting a new job that requires a gazillion hours a week? How can we stave off the afternoon slump that inevitably hits at 3 p.m., leaving us in desperate need of a catnap? Can we create a healthy balance between eating at home and trying the city's newest hot spots; going to the gym after work and unwinding with friends and a glass of wine; cooking in to save money and ordering out to save time?

I want to provide a tool for professional women to achieve their goal of a balanced lifestyle. Feeling good and energetic and yes, having that slim body you've always wanted is achievable, and without making drastic life changes or feeling deprived.

The crux of *The Daily Fix* is that your everyday eating and physical activity habits matter most when it comes to weight management and a healthy lifestyle. Unlike a diet, you do not go on and then off a habit—you form and adopt it, and it becomes part of your life. It doesn't matter so much if a few times a year you get together with friends and polish off a pint of Ben and Jerry's, or if you need an extra-large chocolate chip cookie when you are PMSing. In fact, enjoying your favorite "junk" foods once in a while is a necessary part of life (says your nutritionist). It is the eating behaviors you engage in habitually that make a true impact on your waistline and ultimately on your health. A smart way to look at this concept is in terms of frequency: It is not just *what* you do, but *how often* you do it. If there are certain foods you eat every single day, let's make sure they are healthy habits. I will focus on what you are doing five days in a row every week rather than your behaviors during the weekend, and further, what you do fifty weeks of the year, not during the two weeks you are on vacation.

The Daily Fix is structured chronologically around your workday schedule, since you naturally spend the majority of your time at your job. I am not going to suggest any hard-and-fast rules that impose strict boundaries on your life, *e.g.,* do not eat any carbohydrates, or drink blended power shakes for all of your meals for two weeks. Rather, I want to use the natural framework of the workday to help you establish a clean and sustainable meal and exercise routine. As working women, many of us have fallen into the same predictable patterns of meal, snack, and physical activity habits—we get to work the same way every morning, eat from pretty much the same selection of foods for breakfast, lunch, and dinner, graze for snacks at about the same hour each afternoon, and do the same workouts week after week. Chances are, you already practice some very good daily habits, which I hope to

The Daily Fix Healthy Habits

◆ **#1:** Fix up your morning drink so you can enjoy it, guilt-free, every day.

◆ **#2:** Start every day with a breakfast regimen that includes both fiber and protein.

◆ **#3:** Aim for a midmorning and a midafternoon snack every day in addition to your three regular meals.

◆ **#4:** Eat a lunch that contains high-fiber, high-water-content foods and a portion of lean protein.

◆ **#5:** If you have a sweet tooth (most of us do), have a "sweet nothing" every day.

◆ **#6:** Drink *up to* one alcoholic beverage per day.

◆ **#7:** Use dining out as an opportunity to eat fish.

◆ **#8:** Make a resolution to cook dinner *at least* once a week.

◆ **#9:** Aim for 7 to 9 hours of sleep per night.

◆ **#10:** Walk at least 30 minutes almost every day and work out 4 to 5 times a week at a higher intensity for at least 20 minutes.

◆ **#11:** Drink water with every meal and throughout the day.

◆ **#12:** Remember, a workday is a workday regardless of where you are. Learn to practice *The Daily Fix* while traveling for business.

build upon. But you probably also have quite a few bad ones, which we will try to reduce in frequency. In short, we will target and fix your workday routine to combat the common, unhealthy patterns that often lead to weight gain and low energy in women our age.

I have devised a list of healthy habits for you to incorporate into your life, Monday through Friday. These *daily fixes* hold the key to looking better, feeling more energized, slimming down if you need to, and living longer. They are truly a lasting foundation upon which you can build a lifetime of good health.

Some of you might already be comfortable with these habits, while others may find them particularly daunting. For the latter crew, consider this: Patterns of eating and physical activity are learned. Behavior therapy suggests that it takes about three weeks to change a bad habit or to form a new, good one.[1] I will show you how to incorporate these fixes into your workday, and after three weeks, you should find that you no longer crave your former vices and new, healthier habits have taken their place.

My goal is not only for you to make healthy, wholesome eating routine, *but also that you find it to be pleasurable.* I want you to taste the foods that you eat instead of mindlessly scarfing down a bunch of convenient, processed junk or—equally as bad—live a life beholden to iceberg lettuce salads and diet soda. People in their 20s and 30s have the most sensitive palates, so this is a good time to learn to savor your food. Why waste your high palate on a bunch of mediocre fare? Women, in particular, have a more sophisticated olfactory system (for smell and taste) than men, making us even more capable of savoring every morsel (maybe this is also why we are more drawn to the neighborhood bakery than our male counterparts?). Food is something we are faced with every day, and the sooner we figure out how to eat deliciously *and* healthfully, the better off we (and our families) will be, present and future.

The Daily Fix is designed to be an entertaining and educational cover-to-cover read, as well as a quick and handy on-the-go reference guide. Whether you're looking for a quick snack idea, the number of calories in a glass of wine, a nutritional solution to PMS, or a strategy to fit exercise into your busiest day, you can flip open this book and find the answers you're looking for. Welcome to *The Daily Fix,* ladies—I hope you find it enjoyable, informative, and slimming.

PART 1

Basics

CHAPTER 1

No More Excuses

YOU'RE YOUNG, smart, and well informed. So why is it so tough for you to stay fit and healthy? As a nutritionist, I've heard every excuse in the book for packing on pounds. While most of them won't fly with me, I am sympathetic to some of the challenges you face. Becoming aware of the everyday obstacles that can lead to weight gain is fundamental to your weight-loss efforts. We cannot exclusively blame ourselves for all this extra flab; with approximately 65 percent of American adults overweight, there's clearly something unhealthy going on in our culture.

Obstacles

Simply put, our environment is "food toxic." This idea was first presented by Kelly Brownell, director of the Rudd Center for Food Policy and Obesity at Yale University. He contends that our high-calorie, high-fat, low-nutrition food culture is to blame for our country's upsurge in obesity. Easy access to cheap fast food, snack food, and soda, and limited convenient, healthy choices make it difficult for anyone to eat right 100 percent of the time. With this in mind, it is not surprising that our food supply actually makes approximately 3,900 calories available for every American every single day (including our babies).[1] Reread my last sentence. This number is pretty outrageous: It is nearly double the number of calories an average female needs, and nearly eight times the amount a baby would need, which means that far too many empty calories are floating around. Regrettably, our food culture has spread around the globe. Recent reports about Japan, a traditionally slim society, indicate a growing public health problem of obesity due to their new-found access to and appetite for Western foods.[2]

For women in our age bracket, I've identified four major Saboteurs, or ways in which our environment is working *against* us. It's important to be mindful of these so that we can avoid and overcome them.

SABOTEUR #1: The Starbucks Cookie Effect

Healthy eating can be a daunting task when we are overwhelmed by easy access to excess calories tempting us at every corner. Who needs to pick up a half-pound bag of M&Ms at Best Buy?! I just went in for a digital camera. Sugary snack foods like these are placed unassumingly at the checkouts of most chain retail stores, and can be hard to resist when you're tired, haven't eaten dinner, or have worked a long day. Marketing managers call these health bombs "impulse items." I call it sabotage (cue *Mission Impossible* theme song).

Anyway, back to Starbucks. I find it nearly impossible to go into a coffee shop and order just a plain, brewed coffee—and I'm a nutritionist! Why? Because there is always an alluring display of sweet and gooey (not to mention extra-large) treats taunting me as I stand in line. Empty calories are omnipresent, girls. Becoming more aware of these fat traps will help you avoid falling into them.

SABOTEUR #2 : Variety Is the Vice of Life

Historically, and even up through the mid-twentieth century, the food supply of grains, fruits, and vegetables was regulated by nature's four seasons, so choices at any given time were limited. Blueberry pies in December or fresh-squeezed orange juice in February simply weren't options for most people. But our generation has grown up with easy access to any food at any time of the year due to global trade, technological breakthroughs like refrigeration, pesticides, genetically altered seeds, and the growth of the packaged food industry, which is constantly creating new products (primarily made from corn syrup). Studies have shown that the more variety we have access to, the more we'll eat.[3]

Consider, for example, Thanksgiving dinner. You may feel completely full from the turkey and stuffing and sweet potatoes and announce to the table: "I am stuffed and cannot eat one more bite!" while discreetly unbuttoning your pants. But once dessert— a new food option—is brought out, you can't resist sampling three—yes, three—different types of pie . . . topped with homemade whipped cream. Of course, once a year, this sort of food fest is okay. But on a day-to-day basis, having too much variety or choice among *types* of food causes us to overeat. Whether you are

 CHEW ON THIS!

Brian Wansink, executive director of the USDA's Center for Nutrition, studies the mindless food-related decisions we make every day. His 2004 study examined the influence of variety on consumption. Study participants were offered between six and twenty-four different-colored unmixed jelly beans; those who were offered more variety in colors consumed on average twenty-eight jelly-beans compared to twelve consumed by those who were offered the least colors.[4]

choosing from a breakfast buffet or flipping though a six-page diner menu, be aware of the link between variety and overeating.

SABOTEUR #3: The Media's Mixed Messaging Mess

We are bombarded with food advertisements, diet gimmicks, confusing nutrition research, and blatantly hostile physical critiques of celebrities and models. This is especially pertinent to us, as we are the main readers of gossip magazines, where on one page you find an article about a skeletal star who needs to gain weight and on the next there is a feature about a celebrity who, though she looks tiny to you and me, "can't quite take off the baby pounds." Or we read an article about slow, sustained weight loss via diet and exercise that shares a page with an advertisement for diet pills. The messages just don't add up.

A client once told me she read that eating "lukewarm" food was "healthiest" and asked me to do some research. Obviously highly skeptical (but as a nutritionist, never cynical), I checked into it for her and confirmed that there is nothing scientific about this. My client had fallen victim to yet another confusing gimmick invented to make an article about nutrition sound cutting-edge. As nutrition fallacies and the obsession with weight loss continue to drive media headlines, many of us are left feeling confused. Make sure to read your favorite magazines with an informed eye and enjoy them for their entertainment value, not as a source of education.

SABOTEUR #4: The I-Don't-Want-to-Run-into-a-Cockroach-on-the-Sketchy-Staircase Effect

Both indoors and outdoors, our infrastructure is just not set up for pleasant physical activity. In some suburbs, there are no sidewalks, making it difficult to get anywhere without a car. In many cities, bike lanes and running trails are nonexistent, unsafe, or hard to access. And, much of the time, the staircases in our apartment and office buildings are just too risky. They are dark and damp, can be infested with pests, and are clearly not engineered for daily use (I often wonder if I will be able to exit the stairwell once the door closes behind me). It is overwhelmingly convenient to buy a king-sized candy bar, but it is nearly impossible to bike to work or even simply take the stairs. What a conundrum.

Because most American adults do not meet recommended levels of physical activity, attention is being placed on our "built environment" and its effect on human activity patterns. A relevant report by researchers from Rutgers University calls for America to take note of European laws that support pedestrian and bicycling safety via updated urban design, restrictions on motor vehicles in cities, and regulations protecting non-motorists.[5] On a recent trip to Amsterdam, I became convinced of the merits of this system: The bike lanes and walking paths were superb. Another research paper reviewing environmental interventions to promote physical activity encourages the upkeep of stairwells so people can and will use them.[6] We could be doing far better, not only with our food culture, but also in terms of how our environment is set up to promote physical activity.

These four Saboteurs illustrate how our culture facilitates our addiction to a less-than-healthy lifestyle. It is important to realize that we are up against a whole lot. Just being aware of these obstacles will empower you to make more informed—and ultimately healthier—decisions. Walk past that icing-drizzled muffin in the

Savvy Girl Tip

Beware of impulse purchases, of which candy is king. Make a pact with yourself not to purchase food unless you are in a grocery store or a restaurant. When you go to Blockbuster, FedEx, Best Buy, or the drug store, just say no to the candy in the checkout line.

case at Starbucks, read your favorite magazines without getting bogged down in health trend hype, and say "yes" to taking the stairs at work (though maybe bring a buddy the first time).

Excuses

Environmental obstacles that are clearly not your fault are one thing; excuses are another. You didn't think I was going to let you off the hook altogether, did you? One excuse I hear over and over again from clients and friends alike is that their weight gain is due to "bad genes." At times, there is some validity to this, but I like to point out that there was no obesity epidemic in the United States even thirty years ago—and human genetics have not radically evolved in that timeframe. What *has* changed is our food culture, and consequent eating and exercise habits. While your shape may be genetic, chances are your size is not. In reality, only about 10 percent of adults have an inherent predisposition that makes it difficult to lose weight. "Okay," you think, "then why is my whole family overweight?" Typically the reason is because you have all been raised in the same environment with similar food and physical activity habits, not because you all have a gene that makes it harder to lose weight. And you folks who *do* hold that unfortunate gene can also benefit from healthy habits, so read on.

Beyond genetics, the core of most of the bad excuses I hear from my clients is logistical, revolving around scheduling and time management: working too much to care about anything but work, lack of time to eat three meals a day, eating on the run, not planning snacks ahead, no time to exercise, too much booze at night, and midnight binges. As tough as our culture makes it to stay slim, you do have the power to take good care of yourself by investing some time in organizing your daily routine to include smart eating choices and physical activity.

I find it interesting that it is often the high-functioning women who hold great jobs and sustain healthy relationships who do not take the time to plan ahead and actually think about what to eat, when to work out, and how to fit *themselves* into the craziness of the day. Why should our health take a backseat to work when eating and exercise are the fuel that will keep us productive? If you are eating well, are on a routine schedule, and are working out regularly, you will feel better, look better, and be more competent at work. You will not face the day groggy and irritable, rather, you will be prepared for whatever is thrown at you. Remind yourself that your health and well-being should always be your first priority.

In the next chapters, I will show you how to focus on planning ahead so *time management excuses* won't fly with you either.

PROFILE

3 . . . 2 . . . 1 . . . Action

Bree was a segment producer for a morning talk show. Her goal was to work her way up, from behind-the-scenes production to on-air personality—and she was putting in her time. Along the way, she also put on a few extra pounds. In her mind, it was the result of long working hours, a self-described "absolute lack of time to work out," and green room calorie traps. After all, when she was up for a 6 a.m. segment, how could she resist grabbing a banana nut muffin or cherry danish off one of the catering trays? She also blamed "bad genes" for her extra flab—all the women in her family were on the heavy side. She came to me because she thought she would need to take off this extra weight if she ever wanted to be on-screen.

THE SOLUTION

During our first session, Bree laid out every excuse in the book for her extra pounds. It was clear to me that she would only be successful if she was really ready to make eating and behavior changes within the confines of her work environment. One thing I have learned through my practice: If a client is not truly motivated to make behavior changes, she will not successfully lose weight. Bree and I took a brief look at the Stages of Change[7] model to assess her intentions.

Stages of Change

1) **Precontemplation** (there is no intention of behavior change)

2) **Contemplation** (individual is thinking about change but is still resistant)

3) **Preparation** (individual is ready to create a plan of action; goal setting)

4) **Action** (individual acts on newfound goals and behavior is modified)

5) **Maintenance** (individual maintains action phase and reevaluates what is working and what needs further change)

Bree was clearly past precontemplation at this initial session, as she had come to me for nutrition counseling. She seemed to be somewhere in between the contemplation and preparation stages—she recognized her problem and came to me to set some goals, but was still resistant and created a blockade of excuses she had accepted. My plan was to bring Bree into the preparation stage by setting attainable goals, and then into the action phase, where the real progress could be made.

Today Bree is maintaining the action phase and reevaluating her plan when necessary. She has unshackled her health from her excuses and feels ready for prime time.

CHAPTER 2

Information Is Power

IN ORDER TO BUILD healthy habits into your life and properly navigate our toxic food environment, you need to understand the fundamentals: essential nutrients and calories. Nutrition is a twofold challenge, a balance between eating the right, wholesome foods and consuming the right number of calories to prevent weight gain. I want you to come away from this chapter with a sense of your personal nutrition goals, including the types of food to emphasize in your diet and an estimate of your daily calorie budget.

What Are the Essential Nutrients?

When nutritionists talk about *essential* nutrients, we are referring to the substances that cannot be synthesized by the body (at all or in the quantities we need), which must be obtained via our diet. The macronutrients—carbohydrates, protein, and fat—and the micronutrients—vitamins and minerals—are all essential. They are necessary for normal body function and repair and we need to consume all of them just about every day for optimal health. Generally speaking, we should be getting about

50 percent of our daily calories from carbohydrate sources like fruits, vegetables, and whole grain rice, breads, and cereals; 25 to 30 percent of our calories from fat sources such as nuts, olive and canola oils, and avocados; and the remaining 15 to 20 percent of our calories from protein sources such as fish, lean meat or poultry, low-fat dairy foods, legumes, and soy. Below is a quick-reference nutrition guide that summarizes our daily essential nutrient needs:

WOMEN AGED 20–40	
Calories	1,800–2,000
Carbohydrates	300 g
Fiber	25–35 g
Protein	50 g
Total fat	Less than 65 g
Saturated fat	Less than 20 g
Cholesterol	Less than 300 mg
Sodium	Less than 2,300 mg
Calcium	1,000 mg
Folic acid	400 mcg (micrograms)
Iron	18 mg
Vitamin C	60 mg
Potassium	3,500 mg

To get a little more specific, here is a mini review of some important nutrient concepts. Having a grasp of this information will make it easy to choose healthful foods.

Fiber/Whole Grains

For women aged 40 and younger—so I'm talking to *you*, ladies—dietary fiber intake should be about 25 to 35 grams per day *from food*—not from supplements like Metamucil. Research shows that most people fall short of their daily requirement, and only the healthiest eaters tend to meet it.[1] Just as a refresher: Fiber is a complex found in plant carbohydrate foods—whole grain products like brown rice, and fruits and vegetables—and it cannot be broken down or digested. This is one reason we love fiber: It gives bulk and substance to our foods without extra calories. All fiber is eliminated from your body via your feces (yes, poop). There are two main types of fiber:

◆ **Soluble fiber:** Water-soluble fiber absorbs water and forms a gel that slows digestion. Amazingly, this makes us feel full and prevents us from overeating. For example, think about the way soluble oats (in oatmeal) expand and "gel." This will cause very slow movement through the digestive system and result in a feeling of fullness. Foods that contain soluble fiber include oatmeal, beans and lentils, oranges, grapefruits, pears, and Brussels sprouts.

◆ **Insoluble fiber:** On the other hand, water-insoluble fiber remains unchanged during digestion and plays the role of a "scrub brush," picking up cholesterol and other unwanted substances in your system and carrying them out of your body as waste. Examples of insoluble fiber include edible fruit skins or seeds—these go through your body and come out virtually unchanged.

◆ **Whole grains:** Do not confuse fiber with whole grains. Fiber is one part of a whole grain food, but high-fiber bread won't have the same beneficial compounds that a whole grain bread will. To be considered "whole grain," a food must contain the three whole grain components—the bran, germ, and endosperm. The bran is the fiber portion, the germ provides you with a tiny amount of unsaturated oil, and the endosperm contains little nutrient content other than calories. The reason you're always told not to eat white bread is because it strips away both the bran and germ, leaving you with just the white endosperm—just the calories, none of the nutrition. Here is an illustration of a wheat kernel.[2]

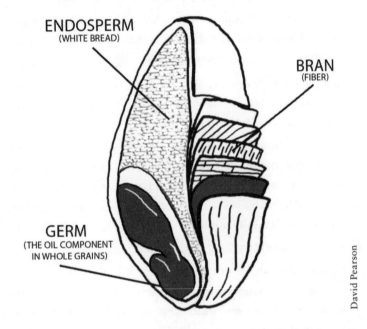

ENDOSPERM
(WHITE BREAD)

BRAN
(FIBER)

GERM
(THE OIL COMPONENT
IN WHOLE GRAINS)

David Pearson

Bottom line: Look for 100% whole grain as the first ingredient, at least 2 grams of fiber per serving when choosing processed foods like bread or rice, and at least 4 grams of fiber per serving of cereal to get the maximum health benefit.

Fat

Very generally speaking, fat derived from animal sources (*e.g.*, whole-milk dairy products, eggs, meat) is saturated and less healthful, while fat that comes from plant sources (*e.g.*, avocados, nuts, and olive oil) is unsaturated and better for you. There's been some controversy about different kinds of fat lately, and you've probably seen trans fats in the news, so I've outlined the basics of what you need to know about each type of fat.

◆ **Saturated fat:** Saturated fats can be found in animal products such as beef, chicken skin, butter, and whole-milk dairy products. Saturated fats should be limited, as they increase your LDL or "bad" cholesterol, which causes plaques to build up in your arteries and, over time, can lead to heart disease (the number-one cause of death in American women). Think of how hard it is to wash away butter from a knife—this is a good illustration of the way saturated fat sticks to your arteries.

◆ **Unsaturated fat:** This type of fat is not saturated with hydrogen so it remains liquid at room temperature. Unsaturated fats, while just as caloric as saturated fats, are heart healthy. They can actually *lower* your LDL cholesterol and increase your HDL, or "good" cholesterol. HDL scavenges our LDL cholesterol plaques for excretion from the body and thus helps to prevent heart disease. This type of fat can be found in vegetable oils, fish, nuts, and avocados. To be more specific:

  ● **Monounsaturated:** Examples include olive and canola oils, avocados, and most nuts (peanuts, cashews, almonds).

  ● **Polyunsaturated:** Omega-3 fatty acids are polyunsaturated and can be found mostly in seafood—more specifically, in fatty fish like salmon, trout, and herring. Flaxseed and walnuts also contain omega-3s.

◆ **Trans fat:** Interestingly, trans fats typically start out as unsaturated fats but then undergo chemical hydrogenation (addition of hydrogen), so they go from liquid at room temperature to solid. Trans fat can be found in vegetable shortenings, some margarines, and processed foods made with partially hydrogenated vegetable oils like baked goods and fried foods. While there is no agreed-upon daily value for trans fats, I recommend you try to keep your trans fat intake as low as possible as it increases your bad LDL cholesterol (like saturated fats do) *but also* decreases your good HDL cholesterol. Look for zero grams trans fat on nutrition labels.

◆ **Cholesterol:** Dietary cholesterol is naturally synthesized by all living things and, as such, is found in meat and seafood. It has little effect on blood cholesterol in most people—rather, it is the saturated and trans fats that affect your blood cholesterol. So, it is a myth that eating seafood like lobster and shrimp—which have dietary cholesterol—will raise your cholesterol. On the contrary, these lean sources of protein have very little saturated fat and include heart-healthy omega-3 fatty acids.

Bottom line: Chose unsaturated fats over saturated or trans fats to get 25 to 30 percent of your calories from fat.

Calcium

Premenopausal women like us should aim to eat 1,000 mg of calcium from diary and nondairy food every day (on top of a possible multivitamin or calcium supplement, to be discussed later with supplements). In a 2007 cross-sectional study of 183 postmenopausal white women, one group got the majority of their daily calcium from supplements, another got it from dairy products and other foods, and a third group got their calcium from consuming both calcium-rich foods and taking supplements.[3] Interestingly, the women relying on dietary calcium (*i.e.*, calcium from food alone) took in the least calcium—on average 830 mg/day—*but* had higher spine and hip bone-density scores than those relying on only supplements, who consumed on average 1,033 mg/day. One explanation is that your body may be able to use dietary calcium more efficiently compared with supplemental calcium. Also notable, but not so surprising, is that women in the diet-plus-supplement group had the highest overall calcium intake at about 1,620 mg/day and tended to have the highest bone mineral density. Premenopausal ladies: Now is the crucial time to make calcium a priority in your diets to stave off osteoporosis and osteopenia in the future, not to mention to save your posture (we all look thinner when we stand up straight!).

Bottom line: To keep your bones as healthy as possible for as long as possible, make eating calcium-rich foods a habit.

5 A Day

By now I'm sure you've heard of the 5 A Day campaign. The Centers for Disease Control (CDC) recommendation is to have *at least* two servings of fruit and three of vegetables every day (but you can always make up for lack of fruit by eating more veggies or vice versa). So, what counts as a serving? One cup of raw, ½ cup of cooked, or ¼ cup of dried fruits or vegetables each typically counts as one serving. Fruits and vegetables are high in water content and thus low in calories; they are high in vitamin C, folic acid, beta-carotene, potassium, and fiber (soluble and insoluble); they can help stave off chronic diseases including some cancers and heart disease; and they can be absolutely delicious. Despite these known benefits, only 40 percent of us are eating five or more ½-cup servings of fruits and vegetables per day.[4] This seems foolish, because filling up on our recommended daily allowance of these foods is one of the simplest ways to stay slim and healthy.

Bottom line: The 5 A Day campaign pro-

Savvy Girl Tip
Make a pact with yourself to focus on your 5 A Day goal. You will find it harder to fit unhealthy foods into your day when you require yourself to eat your fruits and veggies.

motes one of the single best ways to improve your overall health and stay slim—eat your fruits and veggies every day.

Moving on. . . . What Is a Calorie?

Simply put, a calorie is a measurement of energy. Technically, it is the amount of energy or heat it takes to raise one gram of water by one degree Celsius. Macronutrients—carbohydrates, protein, and fat—have calories and thus literally give us energy. Micronutrients—vitamins and minerals—do not have calories, so they cannot give us energy; rather, they put the calories from our macronutrients to work via metabolic reactions.

There are 4 calories per gram of carbohydrate and protein, 9 calories per gram of fat, and 7 calories per gram of alcohol. You may have heard these numbers before, but what do they mean? To give you an idea of what a gram looks like, 1 gram = ⅕ of a teaspoon, so it is a very tiny amount of food. For example, ⅕ of a teaspoon of olive oil, a fat, is about 9 calories, so 1 teaspoon is about 45 calories.

There are 3,500 calories in 1 pound of fat. So, if you decrease the number of calories you eat or increase the number of calories you burn by 500 every day for 7 days, you will lose 3,500 calories, or 1 pound, by the end of the week. Or, you can try to reduce your intake by 250 calories every day for one week to lose half a pound, and so on.

Do I Need to Count Calories?

Most diet plans are either based on counting (*i.e.,* calories, fat grams, or points) or cutting (*i.e.,* whole food groups such as carbohydrates, white foods, or even cooked foods). Of these two strategies to lose weight, I am a proponent of counting calories. It is very important to eat from all three food groups almost every day for optimal nutrition, but you must stay within your calorie budget range (discussed below) for weight management.

So, What Is My Personal Calorie Budget?

Women need approximately 1,800 to 2,000 calories per day to get our essential nutrients without gaining weight. Petite women who are 5 feet tall or less may need fewer calories than this, while women who are taller than 5' 10" may need more. Likewise, very active women may need 2,400 or more calories a day to sustain good health, while sedentary girls may need only 1,400 or fewer calories.

To give you a better idea of your personal calorie budget, you should know your Ideal Body Weight (IBW) range so you can better assess your weight goals. Should you aim to maintain your weight, lose, or gain? Once you figure this out, you can use what nutritionists call the Quick & Dirty Method to get your calorie budget. It takes into account your current weight, weight goals, and physical activity status. Now is the only time when I will ask you to grab a calculator.

Nutritionists calculate Ideal Body Weight for women based on your height using the following formula: 100 pounds for the first 5 feet plus 5 pounds for every additional inch. We take this number plus or minus 10 percent to get your IBW range.

 CHEW ON THIS!

The average weight gain in middle-aged women results from just about 10 extra calories per day over time.[5] This suggests that very small but sustained changes in eating and physical activity behaviors can prevent weight gain. So if you are careful with your calories, you will actually be able to fit into your wedding dress forever.

For example: If Stella is 5' 7" tall, her IBW is 100 + (5 × 7) = 135 pounds; 135 +/− 10% = approximately 120 to 150 pounds.

Depending on Stella's build, she may healthfully fall anywhere in this weight range.

TRY IT FOR YOURSELF

100 pounds + (5 x [how many inches you are above 5 feet]) = ___ pounds

___ pounds +/− 10% = YOUR APPROXIMATE IBW RANGE

Note—In case you want to calculate IBW for one of the men in your life, we use a similar formula: 106 pounds for the first 5 feet plus 6 pounds for every additional inch.

Now we can move on to our second (and final) calculation to figure out your personal daily calorie budget. We will be working in kilograms. To convert your current weight in pounds into kilograms, divide your weight in pounds by 2.2. For example: If Stella is 130 pounds, she is 59 kg (130 ÷ 2.2 = 59). Base your calorie budget on the following criteria:

◆ 40 to 45 calories per kg of body weight to gain weight and/or for intense physical activity (*i.e.*, you are training for an event such as a race or triathlon)

◆ 30 to 35 calories per kg of body weight for weight maintenance and/or moderate physical activity (*i.e.*, 4 to 5 days per week of approximately 30 minutes on the elliptical machine)

◆ 20 to 25 calories per kg of body weight for weight loss and/or low physical activity (*i.e.*, you rarely hit the gym)

So, going back to Stella, if she is looking to maintain her weight and does a moderate amount of physical activity, she should be eating roughly in the range of:

59 kg × 30 calories to 59 kg × 35 calories = 1,800 to 2,000 calories per day as a daily calorie budget range.

You can eat anywhere within your range and be successful, but if you are tall (≥ 5' 8"), you may want to eat on the higher side of this range, while if you are small (≤ 5' 3"), you can try the lower side.

How Do I Determine How Many Calories I Am Eating?

Now that you know how many calories you *should* be eating, it is important to know how to track your intake so you don't overeat. Unfortunately, it's not always easy to figure out how many calories are in your food.

First, it is crucial to estimate portion sizes as accurately as possible. After some time and practice, you may be able to eyeball your portions pretty accurately. But for all new foods—especially for items that are not typically preportioned and can be difficult to assess such as fish, chicken, lunch meat, nuts, rice, cereal, and liquids—it is best to use measuring cups and spoons or a food scale (these are widely available, even at grocery stores) to make sure you are assessing your portions correctly. Here are some easy portion equivalents to keep in mind:

- A deck of cards = 3 ounces of cooked meat
- A checkbook = 3 ounces of cooked fish
- 4 dice = 1 ounce of cheese
- 1 postage stamp = 1 teaspoon of butter
- 1 Ping-Pong ball = 2 tablespoons of peanut butter
- A standard can of soda = 12 ounces of liquid (1½ cups)

Once you know the portion size of the food you intend to eat, you can look up how many calories you are taking in on a food label (discussed further in Chapter 4), in a standard calorie counting reference book, or by searching the huge food database at my favorite free online resource: www. CalorieKing.com.

A rule of thumb: Always round up. *Research has shown that people tend to gravely underestimate both portion sizes and calorie content.* Try to round up to the nearest 50 calories to give yourself some leeway. For example, if you drink what you estimate to be 1 cup of nonfat skim milk, you have ingested approximately 90 calories depending on the milk brand—but if you are unsure of the exact quantity, go ahead and round up to 100 calories. Rounding also makes the math easier to do in your head.

Now that you have a better idea of your personal nutrient and calorie profile, I want to go over some tools of the nutrition trade that will make it easy to track your daily intake. Read on, ladies . . .

PROFILE

The Daily Deal

When Vanessa contacted me for nutrition counseling, it was clear she had a love/hate relationship with her hardcore job as an investment banker on Wall Street. She appreciated the day-to-day challenge and work ethic of her co-workers. She also enjoyed wearing beautifully tailored suits (and the fact that she could actually afford them). The problem was that some of her favorite slacks were feeling a little tight around the waist and she was just too overwhelmed to deal with it while working 15-hour days. Vanessa often forgot to eat breakfast, had only a meal replacement bar for lunch, and would indulge in a big dinner with her colleagues in the conference room or with a client at a steakhouse. She had no idea how many calories she was consuming per day, but she never felt satiated until bedtime, when she was often uncomfortably stuffed.

THE SOLUTION

Vanessa was desperate when she came to me. Because she was a "numbers" woman by nature, she was the perfect candidate to calculate her daily calorie budget to learn once and for all how to keep track of what she ate. Armed with basic calorie-control strategies, Vanessa swiftly lost the extra 7 pounds she had put on. She reports back that she has more energy than ever and she no longer feels bloated at night.

CHAPTER 3

Tools of the Nutrition Trade

YOUR JOB is to make healthy eating a habit. The three tools I introduce here will make this easier. Keeping a food journal will make you more aware of both your typical calorie intake and of the caloric content of your favorite foods. The food frequency questionnaire is designed to show you how often you are (or are not) eating different types of foods. And the calendar, in various forms, is an important tool for maintaining and monitoring your healthy habits.

#1: The Food Journal

Ubiquitous in the practice of nutrition, the food journal is a basic but powerful tool. Now that you know your daily calorie budget, I would like you to journal your food intake for one workweek (five workdays). Though it can be tedious, taking the time to maintain a food journal can also be very effective. The important lesson here is to be able to connect that sandwich you eat every day to its calorie content. You may be shocked to see how caloric some of your favorite foods are or pleasantly surprised to discover those foods that really fill you up are low in calories. And I know you'll be stunned by how many calories are in the bread basket at dinner.

Below is a sample food journal. You can find a blank 5-Day Journal on pages 211–215 for your own personal use (you can even photocopy it and create a month-long journal). Begin each day on a new page and make sure to record EVERYTHING you eat and drink.

To complete a successful food journal:

◆ Column 1: Record the time of day when you eat or drink anything.

◆ Column 2: Describe the food you eat as specifically as possible. For example, do not just write "chicken." Instead, specify white or dark meat, the cooking method used (fried, baked, or broiled), and identify whether it was with or without skin. Another example—specify if your milk is 2%, 1%, skim, or soy, or if your bread is whole wheat or white. Do not forget to include condiments (*e.g.*, butter, ketchup, salad dressing).

◆ Column 3: Record the portion size.

◆ Column 4: Record the calorie content.

◆ Column 5: Record any details you may want to remember: how hungry you felt before eating; how stuffed you felt when you were finished; any digestive issues that might have occurred.

 **CHEW ON THIS!**

After monitoring more than 2,000 dieters who were encouraged to record meals and snacks, researchers at Kaiser Permanente's Center for Health Research determined that the single best predictor of whether a dieter would lose weight was whether the person kept a food journal. The amount of weight each participant lost was directly related to the number of days they kept a log.[1]

Sample Food Journal

TIME	FOOD/DRINK	PORTION	CALORIES	NOTES
7:30 am	Fiber One cereal in skim milk topped with strawberries, orange juice	1 cup cereal 1 cup milk 1 cup berries ½ cup juice	120 cals 90 cals 50 cals 60 cals	Groggy. Watching *Today* show.
10:30 am	Green apple	1 medium	70 cals	Wanted candy but ate apple b/c it was sitting on my desk.
1 pm	Subway Veggie Delite sandwich w/ cheddar cheese; Diet Coke; roasted chicken noodle soup; Dannon strawberry yogurt	6" 2 triangles 12 ounce can 10 ounces 4 ounces	230 cals 60 cals 0 cals 80 cals 110 cals	A great, quick lunch and I got to take a 5-minute walk to pick it up, which felt good.
2:15 pm	Hershey's Kisses—milk chocolate	2 pieces	50 cals	Bored and grabbed off friend's desk.
3:30 pm	Dry roasted, unsalted almonds	1 ounce (16 almonds)	170 cals	In need of a pick-me-up . . . satiating.
8:30 pm	Grilled chicken breast; olive oil; roasted asparagus; brown rice; dry white wine	5 ounces 2 teaspoons 6 spears ½ cup cooked 5 ounces	230 cals 90 cals 20 cals 110 cals 120 cals	Delicious, healthy dinner. Ate with friend and we had a fun time chatting.
10pm	Hot cocoa, sugar-free	1 envelope	30 cals	Craving a sweet . . .

Though I am only prescribing the food journal for one week, feel free to continue until (a) you feel that you fully understand your daily eating habits and (b) you get to the point where you have memorized or can estimate the calories of the foods you typically eat. At the end of the week, review your food journal and ask yourself: "Should I be eating these foods every day, or should some of them be reserved for special occasions?" The goal is to be able to distinguish between good daily choices versus weekly or special-occasion foods, which brings us to our next tool.

#2: The Food Frequency Questionnaire (FFQ)

Along with the food journal, the Food Frequency Questionnaire (FFQ) is a common dietary assessment tool used in large studies of diet and health as well as in one-on-one nutrition counseling. Clients are asked to report the frequency of consumption of different food items over a defined period of time. The idea of the FFQ is to pinpoint food types that might be deficient or excessive in your diet. After you have completed your 5-day food journal, take the time to translate the results into your FFQ. While the food journal helps you convert what you are eating every day into a caloric count, the FFQ allows you to look across the whole week on one page to help you better understand your eating patterns. How many times a week are you drinking a diet soda? Are you getting enough servings of fruits and vegetables over the course of a week? And how many times are you eating dessert? This tool is not about calories; rather, it is about how many servings of a particular type of food you are consuming per day and per week. Your true habits should jump off the page and highlight the strengths and weaknesses of your diet. This exercise will show that there are some habits we should add and maximize—things we should be doing 5 days a week—while others should be reduced in frequency to a weekly, monthly, or even yearly special event.

I have translated the results from the sample food journal opposite into a sample FFQ on the next page. As you can see, I do not get caught up in portion sizes. Though only one day is tracked here, you can imagine how a week's notes will display your eating trends. There is a blank FFQ in the back of this book to record your own results.

SAMPLE FFQ

FOOD	MON	TUES	WED	THURS	FRI	TOTAL/WEEK
Milk	1					
Other dairy products	1					
Fruit	2					
Vegetables	2					
Bread	1					
Rice and other starches	1					
Cereal/granola bars	1					
Poultry	1					
Red meat						
Fish						
Legumes/lentils						
Soy beans/tofu						
Cheese	1					
Eggs						
Nuts	1					
Soup	1					
Olive/canola oil	1					
Butter						
High-fat snacks						
Low-fat snacks						
Desserts/sweets	1					
Juice	1					
Alcohol	1					
Soda						
Diet soda/drinks	2					
Coffee						
Tea						

#3: The Calendar

Last but not least, I want to introduce my favorite tool for working women—one that will provide you with continuous support. And it is at your fingertips—literally. Most likely, you have become all too accustomed to using your mobile device (a.k.a. "crackberry"). But whether you use a BlackBerry or iPhone, Outlook software on your laptop, or a good old-fashioned paper calendar, this ultimate planning tool will make you accountable to your health and fitness. Your calendar can facilitate meal, snack, and exercise scheduling, habit formation, caloric monitoring, and motivation. Here is how to put your planner—electronic or otherwise—to work for your health.

Food

◆ Plan your meals: breakfast, a snack, lunch, a second snack, and dinner, each as a designated appointment on your calendar. At the very least, enter a recurring appointment entitled "snack" just to remind you to take the time during your workday to eat.

◆ Take it one step further: Notate how many calories you aim to consume per eating occasion (calorie ranges are in upcoming chapters).

◆ Consistently track how many calories you actually ingest: This is the easiest way for busy women like us to determine how much "room" is left in our calorie budgets at the end of the day for dinner, dessert, and/or drinks.

Exercise

◆ Plan your workouts: At the beginning of the week, make each session an appointment with a set time. These time slots

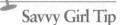

Savvy Girl Tip

In order to stick to your workout schedule, learn how to say no to extra hours at work or to another happy hour you don't really want to attend anyway. Making your health a priority from here on out is mandatory.

will appear as "unavailable" on your calendar, so you'll be less likely to double-book or bail out of exercising at the last minute.

◆ Set up a recurring schedule: If your weekly workout routine generally stays the same, your appointments will show up week after week without you having to update anything. It doesn't get much easier than that.

Motivation

◆ Send yourself timed messages of encouragement: Not only will this help you stick to your plans, but it can provide motivation when you need it most. A simple "Stay away from the candy jar! Save those calories for wine on Friday night!" or "Spend 40 minutes at the gym after work, then go home and watch *Grey's Anatomy* feeling terrific!" can go a long way in providing you with the perspective you need to make a good decision for your health.

No matter where you are, your daily planner is never far away. And let's face it—your BlackBerry is much less conspicuous than a journal at a client luncheon.

Reaching your nutrition goals requires awareness, discipline, and healthy choices. These three tools should help improve your awareness and discipline moving forward. Our next chapter will address making the right food choices.

PROFILE

The Diet Soda Diet

Carrie was a public relations consultant for a hip fashion label. She started her job straight out of college, and unlike most of her friends, was still there five years later. The money was only okay, but the perks were fabulous—Carrie got discounts on ridiculously overpriced clothes (which in reality made them only barely affordable). She was also privy to insider information about the hottest sample sales, and best of all, got to borrow couture gowns every now and then for special occasions. In order to fit into all her fashionable frocks, Carrie kept herself stick-skinny by drinking diet soda all day long. Carrie had been brainwashed to believe that skinny was the only way to be when working in haute fashion. She came to see me because her stomach was often upset and she worried that her diet might be the culprit.

THE SOLUTION

When Carrie arrived, I asked her to fill out a food frequency question-naire and it became glaringly obvious that Carrie was drinking way too much diet soda (five to seven cans per day). All the artificial sweetener she had been consuming worried me. Eventually, we got Carrie down to no more than two diet drinks per day. In place of the rest, she now drinks orange- and raspberry-flavored seltzer waters and plain water with lemon and lime juice. She reported that after three weeks of this switch—from diet soda to flavored water—she could not imagine going back to drinking so much artificial sweetener and feels more hydrated throughout the day. Also, she reports less abdominal cramping . . . all those chemicals had been wreaking havoc on her stomach.

CHAPTER 4

Grocery Shopping and Stocking

GROCERY SHOPPING is a healthy habit, but going to the market just isn't as simple as it used to be. On top of our traditional supermarkets, a plethora of high-end grocery stores, specialty stores, and farmer's markets are cropping up everywhere. What's more, the organic trend has made us think not just about what foods to eat, but how and where they are grown or raised. My goal in this chapter is to simplify the whole experience for you and make it as enjoyable as possible.

Effective grocery shopping is the key to healthy eating. As great as it is to have the option of not cooking, my goal is to make sure you *do* shop for and prepare your own food—at least some of the time. I can promise that you will feel better, lighter, and more energetic if you do it the right way. Also, eating in and preparing lunches and snacks to bring to work are cheaper and healthier than always eating out. Here are some strategies that will help make grocery shopping one of the healthiest ways to use your debit card.

Grocery Shopping Tips

◆ Try to make going to the market a low-stress experience. Find a market that you like and go after dinner on weekdays or before 10 a.m. on the weekends, when stores are typically less busy. To make it more enjoyable for yourself, grab a cup of your favorite hot tea, bring your iPod, or invite along a friend or significant other.

◆ Make a list of what you need for the week and try to do one big shop. At the end of this chapter I will give you my recommendations for staple foods that should always have a place in your kitchen. These items will give structure to your shopping list.

◆ Don't go grocery shopping on an empty stomach, especially if you know you are prone to impulse purchasing. Plan to shop after a meal and stick to your list.

◆ Shop for health over value. Just because something is on sale does not mean it is a good deal, especially for your waistline. Instead, get and use your store's savings card—it can end up saving you a lot of moola (to be better spent on a new pair of jeans).

◆ If you dread grocery shopping or you're simply too busy to make the trip, online grocery delivery services can be a great alternative. And to make your life even easier, most online grocery store sites allow you to save your grocery list so you don't have to recreate it each time you shop. On a rainy Sunday afternoon, instead of trekking to the supermarket, you can simply log in to your account to reorder your groceries for the week. This can also help to keep you on track: By reordering from your standard, healthy list, you can't grab that tempting pint of ice cream or box of cookies.

◆ Try to shop the perimeter of any traditional grocery store to purchase wholesome foods (produce, meats, dairy, breads) and control your selection of packaged foods (snack foods, soda, processed meals), which are generally found in the middle aisles of the store.

◆ When you do purchase packaged foods, be a savvy label reader.

Believe it or not, there are *whole books* written about how to read a food label. Isn't it a bit odd that it takes 100+ pages to decipher a list printed on a 2 × 5–inch space? I want you to know what to look for so you don't have to read these books— trust me, you don't want to. Here is a briefing of the most important information you should be able to get from looking at a standard food label.

◆ (A) *Serving Size*—The recommended portion size. All other numbers on the food label are based on this portion. We often eat more than this suggested serving size, which is okay. It is just important to be aware of how many servings you are actually eating when adding up your calories. For example, if a predetermined serving size of white rice is ¾ cup for 160 calories and you decide to eat 1½ cups, you have eaten two servings and 320 calories.

◆ (B) *Servings per Container*—Tells you how many predetermined servings there are in a product. However, it's not always this simple. Think of a standard 16-ounce Snapple bottle; though it seems like it *should be* a single-serving drink, there are in fact two servings per container in this bottle. If you drink the whole bottle, you will get *double* the calories along with all the other nutrients on the label. Some individually packaged cookies (with just one big cookie per pack) are a funky 2.5 servings—this seems very sneaky to me.

◆ (C) *Calories*—After deciphering both the *Serving Size* (A) and the number of *Servings per Container* (B), look to *Calories* (C) to figure out how much energy you will be ingesting from your food.

Nutrition Facts

Serving Size   (A)
Servings Per Container   (B)

Amount Per Serving

Calories 0   Calories from Fat 0   (C)

	% Daily Value*
Total Fat 0g	0%
Saturated Fat 0g	0%
Trans Fat 0g	
Cholesterol 0mg	0%
Sodium 0mg	0%
Total Carbohydrate 0g	0%
Dietary Fiber 0g	0%
Soluble Fiber 0g	0%
Insoluble Fiber 0g	0%
Sugars 0g	
Protein 0g	

(D)

Vitamin A 0%   •   Vitamin C 0%

Calcium 0%   •   Iron 0%

Phosphorus 0% • Magnesium 0%

* Percent Daily Values are based on a 2,000 calo-rie diet. Your daily values may be higher or lower depending on your calorie needs:

		Calories:	2,000	2,500
Total Fat	Less than		0g	0g
Sat Fat	Less than		0g	0g
Cholesterol	Less than		0mg	0mg
Sodium	Less than		0mg	0mg
Potassium			0mg	0mg
Total Carbohydrate			0g	0g
Dietary Fiber			0g	0g

Calories per gram:
Fat 0   •   Carbohydrate 0   •   Protein 0

INGREDIENTS: Whole Wheat Flour, (Stone Ground Whole Oats, Hard Red Winter Wheat, Rye, Long Grain Brown Rice, Triticale, Buckwheat, Barley, Sesame Seeds), Malted Barley, Salt, Yeast, Mixed Tocopherols (Natural Vitamin E) for Freshness.   (E)

◆ (D) % *Daily Value*—Tells you the percentage of each nutrient (fat, cholesterol, sodium, carbohydrate, dietary fiber, protein, and vitamins and minerals) you are getting per serving based on a 2,000-calorie diet. The % *Daily Value* can be assessed using the following rules of thumb:

- The FDA considers 5 percent of daily value or less to be a low source of that nutrient, and 20 percent of daily value or more to be a high or good source of that nutrient.

- Look for foods with high percentage daily values of fiber, protein, and vitamins and minerals, and low percentage daily values of saturated fat, cholesterol, and sodium.

- It is important to note that these % Daily Values (D) are based on the predetermined Serving Size (A), so if you eat three servings, the percentage daily value will triple—it can become a nutrient-dense source very quickly when the serving size is increased.

◆ (E) *Ingredients*—The first item in the list of *Ingredients* (E) is the most important, as it is the main ingredient found in the product. The rest of the ingredients are listed in order of descending weight, so the second and third items are likely prominent ingredients as well. In our example, the main ingredient is whole wheat flour, but malted barley and salt, the next two listed ingredients, are also important components of this food.

- It is best to avoid eating processed foods with a long list of ingredients (particularly if they sound like they were concocted in a lab). If you cannot pronounce an ingredient, should you be eating it?

- Some common ingredients to avoid (especially if they are at the top of the list) include: anything with the word *hydrogenated*, refined flour (means fiber component of wheat is removed), corn syrup, sugar, and artificial coloring, flavors, and sweeteners.

Health claims

Promises such as "High in Fiber," "Low in Sodium," or "Heart Healthy" are known as "health claims." They are not found on the food label; rather, they are typically displayed prominently on the front of the package. These claims can sometimes be misleading. Make your own conclusions by carefully reading the ingredients and looking at calories, serving sizes, and the percentage daily values of nutrients.

◆ Health claims are based on predetermined serving sizes—so a food that is labeled "Low in Sodium" may actually become high in sodium quickly if you eat a larger portion than the serving size.

◆ The claims I am always happy to see are "Fresh," which means refrigeration is required, and "Locally Grown," which means the product travels one day or less from point of production to point of purchase.

Whole Foods Is the New Neiman Marcus

It is increasingly hip to be a "foodie." Fine wines, local cheeses, and seasonal organics are the newest luxury items. This trend is in part a reaction to increased awareness about the processed food industry as well as a return to quality and taste over convenience and low cost. But it can be a little difficult to know when it is really worth spending a few extra dollars. Let's review some of the newfangled terms and trends proliferating up and down the grocery aisles.

Enviro-Buzzwords

◆ **Organic:** Organic farming refers to produce grown without the use of pesticides, herbicides, or chemical fertilizers, which are routinely used in conventional farming to increase crop yields. For meat, organic means that the animal was raised without growth hormones or antibiotics, which are used in conventional farming to maximize animal growth and reduce the spread of disease. In some cases, organic foods pack in more nutrients than conventional ones do for the same number of calories due to superior soil integrity (for produce) and organic and non-genetically modified animal feed (in the case of meat and dairy).

◆ **Local foods:** Foods with this label have traveled the shortest possible distance from farm to table. The definition is flexible, but usually refers to local, farm-raised fare that travels no more than 150 miles, or a day's worth of driving, to be sold for consumption. Local foods obviously depend on the climate in which you live and thus are typically seasonal and super fresh. They may also taste better than conventional foods, which often have to be picked before they are ripe to

 CHEW ON THIS!

The organics movement has certainly evolved, from a hippie keenness for natural foods stores in the 1960s to a yuppie obsession with Whole Foods to a mainstream "organics for everyone" Wal-Mart–endorsed trend. Between 2001 and 2004, the number of certified organic farming operations in the United States has increased 64 percent.[1]

survive travel and storage before being put on the grocery shelf. You can feel good about purchasing local foods as it helps support your local economy and is typically better for the environment, as less fuel for transport reduces carbon emissions.

◆ **Farmers' markets:** These are typically outdoor markets that feature local, seasonal, and organic produce, meats, and dairy products. They are usually a great source for organic foods at lower prices as farmers sell directly to the public, without going through a middleman.

◆ **Pesticide-free:** This label indicates that food was grown without the use of pesticides, though is not necessarily 100 percent organic. This is a good label to watch for: When you buy pesticide-free foods, you won't have to worry about ingesting chemicals along with your fruits and veggies.

◆ **Free-range, free-roaming:** Animals (such as cows and chickens) raised under free-range conditions have access to the "outdoors." Unfortunately, this term can be misleading because the requirements are vague for this designation. The "outdoors" may mean anything from a grassy pasture to a concrete deck, and "access" can mean animals are outside all day or not at all.

◆ **Cage-free:** More specific than free-range, cage-free hens have the run of a large indoor space; conventional hens are typically caged tightly together. This is a good label to watch for if you are concerned about the humane treatment of animals.

◆ **Grass-fed:** Grass-fed cattle actually graze in a pasture and enjoy their native bovine diet. They are not fed grain and soy from a feed lot (which cows often have trouble digesting and which leads to the use of antibiotics). Typically, grass-fed beef is lower in fat, saturated fat, and cholesterol and higher in antioxidant vitamin C and beta carotene, making grass-fed beef a good call when available.

◆ **Hormone-free:** This term means that the product is from an animal that has not been injected with hormones. An estimated two-thirds of American cattle are injected with hormones to make them grow faster and increase milk production.[2] A genetically engineered hormone, rBGH, is commonly given to conventional dairy cows. Organic cattle cannot be given growth hormones, though hormone-free cattle are not necessarily organic. Always look for this label on dairy foods.

◆ **Heirloom:** Unlike commercial varieties, heirloom vegetables are grown from a "parent" seed which, true to the term, has been passed down through generations. Farmers who grow heirloom crops help to preserve diversity by growing unique fruits and vegetables. Try heirloom tomatoes or peaches— they are delicious.

◆ **Heritage breeds:** Heritage means to meat what heirloom means to produce. In the U.S., the meat industry's priority is to breed animals that gain weight quickly, which has led to the extinction of numerous animal breeds. Heritage animals are hardy and can survive harsh environmental conditions without temperature-controlled buildings and antibiotics. Farmers who breed heritage animals are helping to preserve these genetic traits from extinction.

◆ **Community-Supported Agriculture (CSA):** CSAs are comprised of a community of people who jointly share the costs of a farm operation. In return, they own shares of that farm and receive a weekly or monthly allotment of produce during the growing season. Besides CSAs, many farms offer produce subscriptions, offering weekly or monthly shipments of produce, flowers, or eggs to your home.

- **Fair trade:** This is a social movement that advocates the payment of a "fair" price in exchange for goods, namely exports such as coffee, tea, and sugar from developing countries. You pay a premium price so the growers can make a reasonable living.

- **Fortified with omega-3s:** This label typically refers to eggs produced by chickens that are given feed supplemented with omega-3s. Though the actual amount of omega-3s in these eggs is not monitored, these can be a good option for those of you who don't mind spending a couple extra bucks for breakfast.

Savvy Girl Tip

Make grocery shopping fun, not a chore. Find your local farmers' market and enjoy walking through the different stalls and stands. Along with the items on your list, pick up some fresh flowers to help boost your mood all week long.

- **Farmed vs. wild salmon:** Farmed fish are fed pellets made up of fish parts not fit for human consumption. Studies show that this feed contains more concentrated amounts of polychlorinated biphenyls (PCBs)—toxins from environmental pollutants that may cause cancer—than the feed wild or free-range salmon find for themselves. Thus farmed salmon is more contaminated than wild. The general recommendation is to eat farmed salmon only about twice per month and to eat wild salmon up to eight times in a month. The problem is that wild salmon can be twice as expensive as farmed, and in my opinion, does not taste as good. To diminish PCB content in both farmed and wild fish, clean your fish by removing the skin and the fatty brown part right under the skin before eating—this is where most of the PCBs are. If you do this, it should be safe to eat farmed salmon once a week.[3]

- **Mercury:** You've probably heard a lot of scary stuff in the news lately about mercury and fish. Mercury is an industrial toxin that unfortunately infiltrates our waters and, as a result, gets consumed by our fish. That said, in 2007, the Institute of Medicine (IOM) put out a review that concludes that the benefits of consumption of fish far outweigh any risks from mercury. In fact, the newest recommendations urge all people, including women who are pregnant or of child-bearing age, to eat a minimum of 12 ounces or 2 to 3 servings of fish per week in order to ingest sufficient amounts of omega-3s. The only caveat: Avoid shark, swordfish, tilefish (a.k.a. golden bass), and king mackerel (not Atlantic mackerel). These large fish eat smaller fish and thus contain the highest levels of mercury. White or albacore tuna, which often ends up on this short list, does have more mercury than light canned tuna, but all people can safely enjoy about 6 ounces (approximately two servings) per week.

I understand that organic foods can be expensive and are not always available. Further, we are still studying the impact that broad-based organic farming has on our environment. Is it really better for our soils than conventional farming? Is it a sustainable way to feed the six billion inhabitants of this planet? It is a very complicated issue and not a forgone conclusion that organics are always superior. And it is more critical for some foods to be raised organically than others. With this in mind, I've created a list of the foods I think you should try to buy organic (or not).

◆ **Fruits and vegetables:** The Environmental Working Group (EWG), a research organization in Washington, D.C., has developed a list called the Dirty Dozen. These are the fruits and vegetables that tend to be doused with pesticides that are hard to wash off, or are not typically peeled to discard pesticide-laden skins. So, if you're going to spend on organics, try to buy the following produce: apples, bell peppers, celery, cherries, imported grapes, nectarines, peaches, pears, potatoes, red raspberries, spinach, and strawberries. Always wash produce thoroughly in warm water.

- **Dairy:** I strongly suggest that you eat organic dairy foods. As I mentioned above, nonorganic dairy cows are often treated with growth hormones to produce more-than-natural quantities of milk. This can make the cows sick, so they have to be given large doses of antibiotics. As a result, the consumption of conventional milk has been associated with antibacterial resistance in humans.[4] At the very least, purchase milk labeled "without artificial growth hormones" or "no rBGH." Other benefits of organic milk include longer shelf life (it will last longer in your fridge) and a richer taste because of the natural feed organic cattle receive. It is the best way to go.

- **Meat and fish:** As with dairy, you minimize your exposure to growth hormones and antibiotics by choosing organic meats and poultry. However, don't waste your money buying organic seafood. Organic standards for seafood have not yet been set by the USDA. Right now, both farmed and wild fish can be labeled organic, despite the presence of mercury and PCBs in the water.

- **Baby food:** While this may only be pertinent to some of you, I did want to note the importance of buying organic baby food. Because baby food is often made up of condensed fruits and vegetables, it is a potential source of concentrated pesticide residues. Furthermore, babies' developing systems are especially vulnerable to toxins from pesticides as well as hormones and antibiotics.

- **Packaged food:** There is no reason to buy organic cereals and snack foods unless you like the product. In fact, these foods are not fortified with vitamins and minerals the way conventional foods are, so you will not get as much iron or folate, for example, from an organic cereal as you will from a conventional one. Just something to consider.

Grocery List

Now that you know how to shop, here is a list of foods that should always be in your kitchen, no matter where you choose to buy them: *These are your standard grocery lists for good health.* Having these foods on hand will give you ample meal and snack options, for home and work.

Stock Your Pantry

- ☐ Cereal (without cartoons on the box; try for at least 4 grams of fiber per serving)
- ☐ Old Fashioned Quaker Oats oatmeal
- ☐ Wheat crackers
- ☐ Brown rice
- ☐ Whole wheat pasta
- ☐ Tomato sauce (check the ingredients—you want a sauce made with only tomatoes, olive oil, and spices—no corn syrup or sugar added)
- ☐ Canned diced or whole peeled tomatoes
- ☐ Canned tuna and/or salmon packed in water
- ☐ Low-sodium canned soups (such as Campbell's Healthy Request or Amy's)
- ☐ Canned beans (chick peas, pinto, black, kidney, etc.)
- ☐ Basic seasonings: salt, pepper, brown sugar, Old Bay, taco seasoning, hot sauce like Tabasco, balsamic vinegar, red wine vinegar, low-sodium soy sauce
- ☐ Healthy oils like extra virgin olive oil, canola oil, and nonfat cooking spray (keep oils out of the sun, in a cupboard, so they do not get rancid)
- ☐ Low-calorie hot chocolate packets
- ☐ An assortment of teas

- [ ] Granola bars, LaraBars, or Luna Bars
- [ ] Dried fruit
- [ ] Fruit leathers
- [ ] Bananas (for a bowl on the counter)
- [ ] Avocados (when available)

Stock Your Refrigerator

- [ ] Fruits and veggies galore (including staples of apples, oranges, lemons, lettuces, tomato, cucumber)
- [ ] Nonfat/low-fat milk
- [ ] Nonfat/low-fat yogurt or cottage cheese
- [ ] Calcium-fortified orange juice
- [ ] Eggs
- [ ] Nuts—almonds, walnuts, or cashews, roasted and unsalted (remember, nuts are fats and will go rancid if they are not stored in the refrigerator)
- [ ] Natural nut butters—almond or peanut
- [ ] Hummus
- [ ] Low-fat cheese: reduced-fat cheddar, part-skim mozzarella, or reduced-fat string cheese sticks
- [ ] A block of good parmesan cheese (so much better than pre-grated)
- [ ] Firm tofu
- [ ] Extra-lean turkey bacon (approximately 20 calories per strip, 1 gram of fat or less, and 3+ grams of protein)
- [ ] Whole wheat English muffins
- [ ] Butter alternative (nonhydrogenated and without trans fats)
- [ ] Mustard
- [ ] Salsa (try to buy fresh salsa whenever possible)
- [ ] Dark chocolate Hershey's Kisses or a bar of really good 70 percent cocoa chocolate

Stock Your Freezer

☐ Whole wheat sliced bread (with at least 2 grams of fiber per slice and less than 100 calories)

☐ Frozen veggies (broccoli, spinach, peas)

☐ Frozen fruit (raspberries, strawberries, blueberries)

☐ Ground turkey

☐ Skinless chicken breasts

☐ Frozen cooked shrimp

☐ Frozen meals (to be discussed in Chapter 12)

☐ Pre-portioned low-calorie ice cream treats

☐ Coffee beans

Throughout *The Daily Fix* I will reference the above foods, showing you when to eat them or how to use them when cooking. If your favorite foods are not on my lists, they are likely special-occasion foods. And, if you have small children, don't let them sucker you into buying excess amounts of treats or processed foods. Allowing junk food to be a staple in your household isn't a healthy habit for you, and it isn't a healthy habit for your kids, either.

Okay—we've made it through the fundamentals of Part 1. Next, I'll provide you with a daily plan that synthesizes good nutrition into your real life. Remember, it is your everyday habits that will make a difference to your health and your waistline, and these are what we will target and fix. Get ready for the workweek.

PROFILE

Grocery Shopping Redesigned

When Liz had her first baby, she transitioned her job as a graphic designer from full-time at the office to part-time at home. She hired a nanny to cover her working hours and spent the other half of the week with her new daughter, whom she adored. However, Liz was frustrated by her inability to consistently find time to get to the grocery store. (And, incidentally, her daughter's car seat didn't fit into the grocery carts at her supermarket—how lame.) When Liz worked full-time outside of the house, she ordered take-out for lunch with co-workers and just went to the grocery store on her way home from work and bought food as needed. But, in her work-at-home-mom scenario, not only was Liz home for breakfast, lunch, dinner, and snacks, she also had her daughter (and the nanny) to think about. She needed to be able to stock her kitchen with healthy foods so she could focus on the rest of her life.

THE SOLUTION

When I met with Liz, we immediately went to work on making a weekly grocery list to keep her cupboards, refrigerator, and freezer stocked with healthy foods. I wanted to make sure that she always had something to grab for lunch and snacks, or to prepare for dinner. I also suggested an online grocery delivery service to Liz. Today, she has refined the perfect weekly shopping list for her family's needs, and it is saved online. She logs in to her account and reorders these healthy foods every Sunday, in preparation for the week ahead. Liz reports that she is as busy as ever, but that her kitchen is well-stocked and groceries are no longer a problem.

PART 2

Morning

CHAPTER 5

Caffeine Routine

WELCOME TO MONDAY MORNING, LADIES—the pleasure of Sunday night HBO is seven days away and the workweek lies ahead. There's only one thing that can draw you out of your warm bed: caffeine. But will it come from Starbucks or Dunkin' Donuts? Is it coffee or espresso, green tea or herbal? Will you go for decaf or high-octane, piping hot or over ice? Will it be prepared with skim milk or half-and-half, and should you choose sugar or artificial sweetener? When it comes to your morning fix, the choices are endless. Today it is not uncommon to find three different coffee shops, all within a couple blocks of each other, no matter where you live. You may have a favorite spot—because you prefer the taste, price, or atmosphere there. Or maybe you make your own coffee at home (it's a bargain). You probably also have a favorite drink—a personalized combination of the elements mentioned above. The question is: Have you concocted a healthy habit or a noxious fix? I hope to help you establish our opening Healthy Habit #1: Fix up your morning drink so you can enjoy it, guilt-free, every day.

Is Coffee Good for You?

Many people don't know whether coffee (plain or dressed up in an elaborate drink) is healthful or not. This is because there has been a ton of conflicting research over the years that seems to demonize coffee and caffeine. What we now know is that most people can safely consume about two to three 8-ounce cups over the course of a day. Caffeine acts as a stimulant to the central nervous system, and in moderation inspires increased alertness, greater attention span, and improved energy, as well as slight mood elevation—qualities that should not be discounted.

In addition to the caffeine boost, there are plenty of other health benefits to be imbibed along with your morning drink. Studies show that regular coffee drinkers benefit from its natural antioxidants, which may protect against premenopausal breast cancer, liver cancer, and type 2 diabetes in young and middle-aged women.[1,2,3] Coffee has actually been deemed the number-one antioxidant in the American diet by researchers who estimate that we get more antioxidants from coffee than any other dietary source[4] (though that statistic should probably be taken with a grain of salt, since coffee is more widely consumed than other antioxidant-rich foods, such as fruits and vegetables). Research has also shown an association between drinking coffee and decreased risk for Alzheimers and Parkinson's diseases.[5,6] Of course, coffee's more immediate

 **CHEW ON THIS!**

An antioxidant is a dietary substance that prevents free radicals (found in cigarette smoke, exhaust from cars, pesticides, etc.) from breaking down healthy cells by bearing the brunt of the breakdown themselves.

impact is the stimulation of the gastrointestinal tract, producing a laxative effect that can send you running to the restroom within minutes of taking your first sip. As long as this does not irritate your stomach, it can be a real benefit toward reducing constipation and helping to keep you on a regular, ahem, schedule.

That said, coffee might not be a good choice for you if you have high blood pressure, a sensitive stomach, or it makes you feel jittery or nervous. Research has also indicated that drinking *unfiltered* coffee (e.g. boiled or French press) is associated with elevated cholesterol levels, likely due to two lipids (*i.e.,* fats)—cafestol and kahweol—that are found in coffee grounds. [7,8] So, on a daily basis, try to stick to filtered (drip) coffee.

I also want to set the record straight about the association between caffeine intake and the risk of osteoporosis. The bad news is that caffeine can be hard on your bones. In a 10-plus-year retrospective study of nearly 32,000 middle-aged Swedish women, daily intake of 320 mg of caffeine (about four cups of coffee) was associated with increased risk of osteoporotic fractures, especially in women with low calcium intakes. [9] It is clear that the more coffee a woman drinks, the more calcium is excreted in her urine. The good news is that this loss is minimal—it only takes about 2 tablespoons of milk or yogurt to replace the lost calcium for each 8-ounce cup of coffee you drink. Furthermore, intake of milk (preferably nonfat or low-fat) in your coffee will count toward your daily calcium requirement if it is more than just a couple of tablespoons.

Finally, it is important to note that coffee does have a mild diuretic effect (*i.e.,* it makes you pee). But for the most part, this loss is compensated for by its water/liquid content—so drinking coffee shouldn't dehydrate you as long as you don't overdo it. If you're drinking more than three cups a day, though, try to increase the amount of water you are drinking.

How Much Caffeine
Is in My Coffee?

Most people think that there is more caffeine in espresso than in regular brewed coffee. Ounce for ounce, this is true. One ounce of coffee has between 10 and 25 mg of caffeine whereas 1 ounce of espresso contains roughly twice that, approximately 30 to 50 mg of caffeine. However, a portion of coffee is typically at least 8 ounces (1 cup) and has approximately 60 to 180 mg of caffeine, whereas a typical portion of espresso is only 1 or 2 ounces (and to that you may add hot water or steamed milk). So, per serving, espresso shots and drinks actually contain *less* caffeine than coffee drinks. Both options can be healthy in moderation, and when plain ("black") contain no real calories—fewer than 5 per serving—so these drinks are easy on the waistline.

By the way, if you're a decaf drinker, you should know that most decaffeinated coffee does contain some caffeine. In fact, a study from the *Journal of Analytical Toxicity* proved that consuming four 16-ounce cups of decaf throughout the day could cumulatively result in the consumption of almost 60 mg of caffeine, the amount found in a cup of the real stuff.[10]

Is Tea a Healthier
Choice than Coffee?

Today, tea is practically as popular as coffee and can be found in at least as many brands and varieties. You have likely tried a few basic types of tea—oolong, black, green, white, and herbal. Oolong, black, and green teas all come from the same tea leaves, but vary in flavor due to how long the leaves are exposed to air oxidation. Black tea is exposed to air for up to 4 hours, green tea is not oxidized at all, and oolong teas is somewhere in the middle. White tea comes from the same leaves as the others, but is picked when the leaves are still just buds and covered by fine, white hair. Herbal teas, on the other hand, come from the roots, stems, flowers, seeds, and leaves of non-tea plants and are not technically tea at all. Chamomile, ginseng, and echinacea are popular herbal teas.

There has been a lot of buzz recently about the supposed anti-cancer and weight-loss benefits of tea, especially green tea. Though more studies are necessary to determine how tea impacts health, it is true that both green and black teas contain polyphenols, which are substances that have been shown to act as anti-oxidants. That said, you'd have to drink a substantial amount of tea (well over five cups a day) to reap potential cancer-fighting advantages. So, go ahead and drink as much hot or iced green and black tea (without cream and sugar) as you like and can tolerate.

Savvy Girl Tip

If you enjoy your coffee while on the road, invest in a coffee mug with a lid that fits into your car cup holder. Help save a few trees by asking your barista to fill your mug each morning instead of using a paper cup.

One caveat: Try to steer clear of bottled iced teas touting an excess of health benefits—they likely contain either tons of sugar or artificial sweeteners and flavors. Try preparing your own unsweetened iced tea at home in a traditional kettle, or make "sun tea": Steep two teabags in a glass jar with about 6 cups of water and put it in the sun for at least half an hour, then refrigerate. Put your homemade iced tea in a reusable water bottle, and you are good to go for the day.

In terms of caffeine content, caffeinated tea does contain slightly less caffeine than caffeinated coffee. An 8-ounce cup contains anywhere between 20 and 110 mg of caffeine (as we have already established, an 8-ounce cup of coffee contains 60 to 180 mg of caffeine). This wide range results from the length of time you let your tea steep, and the variety and size of the tea leaf. On its own, tea is also calorie-free and so is a great option to keep you feeling full between meals.

Bottom Line—How Do I Create a Healthy Daily Drink?

Now that you know the health benefits of your morning brew, let's look at some of the good—and bad—options for your healthy habit. Try any of the following drinks as an everyday fix. Just make sure to order a small (8- to 12-ounce) or medium (14- to 16-ounce) size and ask for skim or low-fat milk. Most coffee shops use whole or 2% milk as a default, so you must specify your choice. You can also request organic or soy milk at select cafes.

◆ Regular or flavored brewed coffee (black)

◆ Espresso

◆ Americano (espresso shot with hot water)

◆ Misto or café au lait, with skim milk (half regular coffee, half steamed milk). This is *my* daily fix!

◆ Latte with skim milk (a shot or two of espresso that has been poured into a cup filled with steamed milk and then topped off with foamed milk)

◆ Cappuccino with skim milk (usually one-third espresso, one-third steamed milk, and one-third foamed milk—more foam than a latte)

 CHEW ON THIS!

Many folks go gaga for Starbucks—I am guilty as charged. But some find the coffee to be too strong. Get this: Starbucks is such a huge company that they must source their coffee beans from all over the world. In order to make their drinks taste uniform in flavor, they blend and (over-) roast these assorted beans.[11] This gives their coffee a very strong, even burnt quality. Furthermore, because many of their drinks are made with excess amounts of milk and sugar, weak coffee would get lost in the mix. Just a little food for thought.

- Macchiato with skim milk (an espresso with a small amount of steamed milk on top)

- Teas (black, green, white, or herbal teas; hot and iced)

Desk drawer staples

Keep a variety of your favorite teas stashed away. Go for caffeinated green tea or spicy chai for a pick-me-up and decaf orange or jasmine for a sweet-tasting, non-caffeinated, calorie-free treat.

When it comes to sweetening your drink, try using just 1 teaspoon of real sugar (the amount in one packet of Sugar in the Raw)—it is only 20 calories. By moderating the amount of real sugar you use, you can reduce the calories and forget the chemicals that come with artificial sweeteners. Also try adding a sprinkle of the spices available at many coffee shops, such as cinnamon or nutmeg, which will add sweetness and flavor to your favorite brew without any calories.

Extras to Avoid on an Everyday Basis

- Artificial sweeteners—Splenda, Sweet 'N Low, and Equal can be found at almost any coffee shop. While these are crucial for diabetics, calorie-free, high-intensity sweeteners may actually increase our appetites for ultra-sweet foods. Plus, there is ongoing controversy regarding the link between artificial sweeteners and increased cancer risk. While the FDA does grant GRAS (generally regarded as safe) status to sweeteners, I would control intake of nonnutritive sweeteners to two drinks per day (for example: a packet of Equal in one coffee and one can of Diet Coke). Remember, you are what you eat.

- Whipped cream—ask your barista to "hold the whip" and you will save anywhere between 60 and 110 calories and 7 to 10 grams of fat!

- Cream and half-and-half—try to use low-fat or nonfat milk instead, or simply use 1 to 2 teaspoons of the heavy stuff.

- Flavored syrup—each pump has 20 to 25 calories. This should be a special treat, not a daily habit.

- Mocha—tends to be coffee or espresso with milk and chocolate syrup added. Would you eat chocolate for breakfast *every day*?

- Any drink made with chocolate chips, java chips, white chocolate, or caramel—this is liquid candy.

- Large (20-ounce) or extra large (24-ounce) drinks. These will likely contain too much caffeine, and it is harder to maintain small amounts of milk, sugar, or artificial sweeteners in a drink that size.

If your drink is not on the Good Options list, you should not be drinking it *every day*. Remember, we're focusing on your weekday healthy habits. Once every couple of weeks you can treat yourself to a chai tea latte or a Frappuccino *with* whip—but remember, these drinks are liquid desserts (even the light versions) and should be treated that way. I know how tempting it can be to order something sweet and yummy when you walk into a coffee joint and are hit with that amazing smell. This may be reason enough to skip this ritual altogether and make your own coffee at home (which is also the most economical option). But if going to the coffee shop is part of your morning ritual or a much-needed afternoon break, fix it so you can enjoy it—guilt-free—every day.

All right—we have learned how to make a healthy choice when it comes to one of our most beloved daily fixes. Now that you are out of bed and feeling alert and energized, let's focus on what is really important—food—and more specifically: BREAKFAST!

PROFILE

Chai Won't Fly

Margo was finally living the life she had always dreamed of. After trying numerous jobs she just couldn't get into—fashion PR, ad sales at a women's magazine, event planning—she finally took out a loan and opened up her own clothing boutique. After a year of hard work, Margo's store was profitable and she could not believe that she was making money by indulging in her ultimate fix every day—designer clothing. Margo routinely tried on the new duds that would arrive at her store and modeled them for her employees. Margo had always been a slim girl and a healthy eater. So, you can imagine her surprise one day when she went to try on a new pair of jeans, only to find that she had to go up a waist size.

In thinking it over, the only thing Margo could remotely identify as a big change to her diet was that she had switched from drinking a large black coffee in the morning to a medium chai tea latte . . . with whipped cream. Initially, she tried the chai latte one Saturday afternoon with her sister, but it quickly became a craving and then a daily fix. In her mind, even with the whip, how could one drink a day make that much of an impact on her waistline?

THE SOLUTION

When I met with Margo, we went through her daily eating habits. It quickly became clear that the chai was indeed her fatal flaw. A 16-ounce chai tea latte (prepared with 2% milk by default) with whipped cream ran Margo 310 extra calories per day compared to the 5 calories she had been getting from her black coffee. Over the course of a 7-day week, this was a difference of 2,135 calories, or more than half a pound. Slowly but surely, this minor change took its toll on Margo's weight. I counseled Margo to forgo her daily chai latte and instead enjoy it as a treat once a week. She promptly returned to her former healthy habit—a plain brewed coffee every day—and within a couple months, was back to her natural size. Margo reports that simply becoming aware of the impact one chai a day could have on her weight status was enough for her daily cravings to cease altogether.

CHAPTER 6

I Am What I A.M.

I KNOW YOU'VE probably heard it before, but that's because it's true: Breakfast *is* the most important meal. It is your first shot at laying the foundation for a healthy day. That's why I am dedicating this chapter to Healthy Habit #2: Start every day with a breakfast regimen that includes both fiber and protein.

While there is no one "best" breakfast, starting your day with a little bit of fiber (to get your bowels moving) and a little bit of protein (for sustained energy and appetite control) improves the overall quality of your diet. As a rule, you should be eating in the neighborhood of **300 to 500 calories for breakfast** to set you up with a boost of energy for the day, and fewer cravings throughout.

As a working woman, I know it can be difficult to fit this meal into your hectic morning, so I will highlight strategies and breakfast options that can be incorporated into your busy routine with ease. Here are three typical morning scenarios. Find the one that you most identify with, and decide which tips are helpful to you.

Scenario #1: *You skip breakfast altogether, as you aren't really all that hungry when you wake up, and further, it saves you calories and time.*

Do you skip breakfast to save calories and lose weight?

Your morning meal can actually help you lose weight. The National Weight Control Registry is an organization where people who lose at least 30 pounds and keep it off for at least one year can register. Common threads between these individuals are tallied to see what works for losing weight and keeping it off. They have found that eating breakfast *is a key characteristic* shared by successful weight loss maintainers.[1]

In general, skipping meals slows down your metabolism. After sleeping 6 to 10 hours at night, your body is ready and willing to take in calories and use them for energy when you wake up. If you delay your intake until, say, lunchtime, you are giving your body a message that it may not get fed. Your body panics and decides to hold onto fat stores along with whatever it is that you consume when you eventually get around to eating. This may be a result of the "thrifty gene" we inherited from our ancestors.[2] Unlike us, they did not always have enough to eat, so their bodies became very good at storing calories and slowing the metabolism to adapt to lower intakes. This is why eating on a schedule, and not waiting too long between meals or snacks, will increase your metabolism.

Skipping breakfast is also consistently associated with overeating at the next meal. By the time lunch rolls around, you are so hungry that you want to binge on whatever you can get your hands on, healthy or not. Or, perhaps you rationalize the cheeseburger and fries because you saved calories from not eating breakfast. The research is clear: Breakfast is a pillar of weight management.

   CHEW ON THIS!

Check out the National Weight Control Registry at www.nwcr.ws. You can browse their additional research findings or register your-self if you fit the criteria.

Do you skip breakfast to save time?

You figure you can use those extra 15 minutes that would have been wasted on eating breakfast to get more work done. But did you know that the morning meal has been proven to increase alertness *and* productivity? So with a little food in your stomach, you will actually use your time more efficiently. In fact, research shows that a high-fiber, low-fat breakfast increases alertness all the way until lunchtime.[3] Studies have also indicated that eating breakfast can enhance your ability to manage tasks that require memory.[4] To avoid nodding off at your desk or forgetting your boss's birthday, try some breakfast.

Do you wake up without an appetite in the morning?

If you're not hungry in the morning, take a closer look at your evening routine. Maybe you are a late night snacker (or binger), or you are simply consuming too much for dinner just before going to bed. These scenarios are likely to leave you feeling full when you wake up the next morning. A good strategy to halt your unhealthy evening habits is to concentrate on morning eating. And once you become a breakfast eater, you will likely not be as hungry or feel as inclined to eat late at night. Eventually, like coffee, breakfast can become a powerful motivator to get you up in the morning. I know I go to sleep thinking about what I am going to eat for breakfast, and my favorite cereal unquestionably helps me get out of bed when the alarm goes off.

Scenario #2: *You eat a swift breakfast at home—say, a glass of OJ and a quick bowl of cereal with a splash of milk. You steal bites in between getting dressed, blow-drying your hair, packing your bag for work, and watching segments of the* Today *show.*

Do you rush through breakfast every morning?

It is important to eat mindfully in order to let your brain know that you have had a meal. I suggest that you sit for *at least 5* minutes either at home or at work and just focus on breakfast eating, on how your food tastes, and how you feel eating it. If instead you eat in a frazzled state, your brain may not register that you have eaten a meal's worth of calories. You may feel unsatisfied, and you will be more likely to munch away mindlessly through the morning. Interestingly, in France, where women "don't get fat," meals are meant to be savored and enjoyed. This thin culture celebrates mealtimes and gives food the respect it deserves.

Are juice and cereal healthy breakfast options?

With all the unfavorable publicity surrounding processed foods and liquid calories, are cereal and juice actually good at-home breakfast options? I say yes, but with the following guidelines:

◆ **Juice:** Many of us drink juice as a breakfast habit—orange, grapefruit, apple, or cranberry. Headlines of late have demonized juice as sugar water, indicting it as a main cause of our country's obesity epidemic. I would not go so far as to say that juice is our enemy, but I do believe that control of liquid calorie intake is a mainstay of weight management. There is evidence that our brains actually have a different mechanism to process calories coming from liquid sources than calories that come from solid foods.[5] As a result, liquid calories do not fill us up or satiate

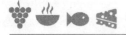 CHEW ON THIS!

Do you know why we call our morning meal "breakfast"? If you have never thought about it before, it will seem commonsensical. When you wake up after a long sleep, your blood sugar is at a fasting level; "breaking that fast" fuels you for the whole day.[6]

us in the same way that food calories do, but it is very easy to drink hundreds of excess calories that will ultimately be stored as fat. Further, it is true that most fruit juice is high in calories, laden with sugar, and lean on nutrition. Think about how many oranges it takes to get a large glass of fresh-squeezed OJ—two, three, four??? Would you eat two, three, or four oranges in one sitting? The phrase "too much of a good thing" applies here. It would be better to eat just one whole orange, apple, or grapefruit than to drink the juice in the first place, as the whole fruit contains fiber that gets filtered when juice is made.

Generally, water is the best accompaniment to all of your meals. But if you love your morning OJ, I recommend a serving of about 4 ounces (which is ½ cup) of 100 percent juice per day. Orange and grapefruit juice are the best options, as 4 ounces can provide you with approximately 60 percent of your daily vitamin C requirement. Also, some orange juice is fortified with calcium, so that is a bonus as well.

◆ **Cereal:** Let's briefly discuss the most popular breakfast food in America—cereal—and how to choose a healthy one from the overwhelming selection on the market. The way that I think about cereal is that it typically provides us with energy (calories), some of our daily fiber requirement, a multivitamin shot due to mandatory fortification of conventional cereal grains, calcium and vitamin D from milk, and—yes—a whole lot of sweet stuff. Unfortunately, nowadays, no matter what cereal you choose, it is bound to contain at least some sugar. I'm not too worried about this generally, as long as you absolutely stay away from *children's* cereals, which

Savvy Girl Tip

All girls know size matters. Swing by your favorite home goods store (mine is Crate and Barrel) and pick up a set of 4-ounce juice glasses to be used in the a.m. to control your liquid calorie intake. It's much easier to regulate the size of your pour with a portion-sized glass.

are loaded with sugar. Sorry, but your days of Froot Loops in the morning are long gone.

Some no-brainer cereal options include "the originals" (which have been on the market for years):

✓ Quaker Oatmeal	✓ Mueslix	✓ Cheerios
✓ Grape-Nuts	✓ Wheaties	✓ Fiber One
✓ Total	✓ All-Bran	✓ Shredded Wheat

Newer to the market, Kashi high-fiber cereals and Barbara's Organic cereals are also healthy and delicious options to try. Remember, you can always mix two cereals for more interesting flavor and crunch. Just make sure to stick to appropriate portion sizes—don't eat double the amount of cereal when mixing. Try to use at least one of my no-brainer options listed above—more specifically, Fiber One is a perfect mixer as it is full of fiber and low in calories. And always be aware of calorie content—some healthy cereals contain a ton of calories—*i.e.*, granola and Great Grains. These are healthy choices only if you stick to appropriate serving sizes or mix them with low-calorie options—Great Grains is delicious with Cheerios.

Remember also to bulk up your cereal by sprinkling it with different toppings. Any fresh fruit is a great choice, including bananas, strawberries, or blueberries—these will increase your breakfast portion and give you antioxidant power without many calories. You can also add a tablespoon of dried fruits like raisins, cherries, or apricots to increase your fiber and iron intake; or a tablespoon of sliced almonds, crushed walnuts, or ground flaxseeds to increase your consumption of omega-3 unsaturated fatty acids, protein, and fiber.

◆ **Milk:** Now, let's briefly discuss cereal's sidekick—milk. If you haven't already, switch to low-fat or nonfat dairy. Milk fat is saturated fat. In fact, though whole milk is recommended for babies under 2 years of age, it is recommended that persons aged 2 and older in this country use nonfat and low-fat milk and dairy products exclusively.[7] If you are lactose intolerant or get gassy and bloated after eating dairy, try low-fat or nonfat calcium-fortified soy milk, Lactaid milk, or take Lactaid pills with your cereal to help digest the lactose in the milk that causes your malaise. Aim for 1 cup of milk in your cereal (8 ounces), as it provides approximately 30 percent of your daily calcium requirement. And make sure to slurp up the leftover milk at the bottom of the bowl!

Scenario #3: *You grab breakfast on your way to work, to be eaten while commuting or to be scarfed down at your desk; a quick stop at your favorite bagel shop, drive-thru, or corner deli will do the trick.*

Do you consistently grab breakfast on the run?

Muffins, donuts, bagels, and greasy breakfast sandwiches have long been in our repertoire of on-the-go breakfasts. The problem is that nowadays, we are constantly on the go and these are not suitable everyday choices. While I'm glad that you actually take the time to get breakfast, a blueberry muffin will not keep you satiated until lunch, as it is all but void of fiber and protein. In fact, most muffins are basically white flour, sugar, and butter (also known as cake), which digest quickly and leave you feeling hungry. Furthermore, they can cost you more than 500 calories while providing few nutrients.

So, what is a *healthy* grab-and-go breakfast for the workweek? Try for a meal that includes both a bit of fiber and some protein to really start your day with a boost that lasts through the morning. Either plan ahead and brown-bag the following breakfast suggestions, or pick them up at your local deli or convenience store on your way to work. Here are some ideas that include both protein and fiber and are well within a calorie budget of 300 to 500 calories.

- A 6-ounce yogurt or low-fat cottage cheese and a granola bar
- A yogurt parfait topped with fruit and granola
- A Luna bar and a whole piece of fruit (try a pear, grapefruit, peach, apple, or orange)
- An Odwalla Superfood Juice Drink and a LaraBar
- An on-the-go bowl of cereal (maybe Special K or Smart Start) with low-fat or skim milk and a piece of fruit
- A packet of instant oatmeal (you can add hot water at work)
- 2 skim or low-fat cheese sticks (think Polly-O) and an apple
- An apple or banana with 3 tablespoons of almond butter
- A peanut or almond butter sandwich (2 tablespoons nut butter) on whole wheat bread and a piece of fruit

How can I improve my breakfast sandwich?

When you are feeling sluggish or maybe a little hazy from too much wine the night before, a greasy bacon, egg, and cheese breakfast sandwich may seem like just the thing to perk you up. I am here to remind you that more often than not, this meal becomes "discomfort" food quickly after you finish it. Who needs a food coma at work? On the weekends, you can eat a fuller brunch meal and then maybe take an afternoon nap. But during the week, you do not have this luxury. Stick to some healthier options to fuel you up without slowing you down. Here are some ways to build a better breakfast sandwich:

Desk drawer staples
Keep a stash of instant oatmeal packets and a box of high-fiber cereal ready to go if you are running late but still need a healthy way to start the day when your arrive at your desk.

- Instead of a bagel, order whole wheat toast. Many bagels pack the caloric equivalent of *more than four slices of bread.*

- Or, try your bagel "scooped out." This literally means that the inside or doughy part of the bagel is dug out and thrown away, leaving you with a much less dense bagel and more like half the calories. While it used to be a New York thing, bagels across the nation are super-sized these days. Enjoy your "scooped out" bagel without the guilt. And order it whole wheat when you can.

- Try egg whites. One whole egg is in the neighborhood of 80 calories, while an egg white has only about 20 calories. Ask for one whole egg mixed with a couple of egg whites—egg whites are surprisingly yummy on their own, especially with some chives, tomatoes, and salt and pepper.

- Add salsa and hot sauce to your egg sandwich. Salsa packs antioxidants and vitamin C with negligible calories, and hot sauce jolts the tastebuds and may create a satiating effect.

- Order light or whipped cream cheese *on the side* so you put it on (in a reasonable portion—2 tablespoons, at most), and top that with tomato and cucumber slices.

- Order a bagel with turkey on it—even for breakfast. The protein will go a long way toward staving off feelings of sluggishness.

- If available, order avocado instead of cream cheese on your bagel. Both are creamy-tasting fats, but avocado is unsaturated and heart-healthy, while cream cheese is saturated and can lead to atherosclerosis. Better yet, ask for avocado on whole wheat toast—it is surprisingly delicious.

- Add some veggies to your morning routine to start the day with a load of nutrients. Order tomato, cucumber, and avocado on your breakfast sandwich, and get eggs cooked with veggies (when available).

I hope you enjoyed breakfast—now it's time to get down to work. I will see you in a few for your midmorning snack.

PROFILE

Breakfast Rx

Eve was the mother of two small children, and held a busy job as a family doctor. In general, her work/life balance was excellent, as she got to do what she loved—practice medicine—and her hours allowed her to spend plenty of time with her family in the evening. It was only the rushed and hectic mornings that made her day stressful. Eve typically woke up early, just before 6 a.m., to get her youngest set up with the nanny, get her oldest to preschool, and get herself to work by 7:30 a.m. Her breakfast was an afterthought, and she would typically get something quick—usually a granola bar—just before running out the door. Eve was usually starving by midmorning and in desperate need of a snack. She would end up grabbing whatever she could get her hands on in the nurses' station or off the reception desk in between patient appointments (usually candy or baked goods).

THE SOLUTION

It was immediately clear to me that Eve needed a breakfast makeover. A granola bar simply was not enough food to keep her satiated from 6 a.m. until noon, and grabbing sweet snacks midmorning to compensate was not healthy or satisfying. Eve needed quick breakfast solutions, as well as healthy snacks to munch on in between patients, to keep her going throughout the morning.

I advised Eve to plan ahead the night before (after her kids were asleep) and pack a portable, easy breakfast. I wanted her to get about 300 to 500 calories with a little fiber and protein. A good choice would be an almond butter sandwich on whole wheat bread with a banana, or a Luna bar and an orange, both of which she could easily throw in her bag at night. For her midmorning snack, I wanted Eve to get about 100 calories, and again, it needed to be something she could throw in her bag on her way out the door. I suggested a yogurt or a baggie filled with dried fruits like apricots or cherries.

Today, Eve is prepared. When she gets to the office in the morning, she eats her preplanned healthy breakfast while taking stock of her patient load for the day. She also carries her midmorning snack in her white coat for easy access. She is less stressed in the mornings and more energized throughout the day.

CHAPTER 7

The Midmorning
Snack Attack

It's 11 A.M. AND—despite eating a healthy breakfast—you're craving a little something and can't wait until lunch. The good news? You *should* have a snack. Let's establish Healthy Habit #3: Aim for a midmorning and a midafternoon snack every day, in addition to your three regular meals. The bad news? You probably start noshing at about this time. You are bored or stressed and mindlessly grab a handful of M&Ms off your assistant's desk, a bagel from the conference room leftovers, a Snapple from the work fridge, or maybe you just start munching on pretzels or whatever your usual fix tends to be. In this chapter, I will discuss how to appropriately satisfy the midmorning munchies.

The Plan

The night before work, plan ahead for **one small snack (no more than 100 calories)** and **one more substantial snack (100 to 200 calories)** for the next day. Your immediate reaction to my last sentence may be "I am way too busy." But let's face it—you spend plenty of mental energy thinking about your weight, obsessing about your body, and planning outfits that are slimming. Why not spend some of that time being proactive?

I suggest that you have your healthy, planned, preportioned smaller snack midmorning, around 11 a.m. I find that before lunch, many working women don't even have time to breathe—too much e-mail, too many meetings, phone calls, etc. Further, if you are eating the breakfast that I call for in Chapter 6, you will probably be generally satiated and won't be starving before lunchtime. This is great because it is even better to munch *before* you feel overly hungry to prevent giving into naughty temptations. Save the larger snack for midafternoon (to be discussed in Chapter 9).

Snacks have many purposes: They keep your blood sugar levels stable between meals, give you a brief boost of energy, prevent you from overeating at your next meal, give your body important nutrients, and snacking brings us pleasure. However, many classic snack foods are processed, full of calories and sugar, and lean on nutrition. If your snack is too sugary, you will experience a temporary peak in energy (a "sugar high") followed by a big crash.

I'd like to mention high-fructose corn syrup (HFCS) at this juncture, as it has become a principal sweetening ingredient in just about every packaged snack food and drink out there. It has replaced sugar because it is a cheaper source of sweetness, largely due to the abundance of corn subsidies in the United States. Currently, HFCS is being researched as a leading cause of obesity and diabetes in this country. In 2007, researchers at the University of Maryland reviewed evidence associating HFCS and weight gain and found that it does not contribute differently than other sources of

---

Desk drawer staples

Bring five whole pieces of fruit to work every Monday to sustain you for the week (apples, oranges, and bananas do not need refrigeration). Keep them in a drawer, or better yet, in a cute bowl on your desk.

---

energy (a calorie is a calorie).[1] However, it is the ubiquitous nature of this sweetener that has no doubt played a role in our overweight culture. Whenever possible, choose foods (particularly packaged snacks) that do not contain this sweetener.

For your midmorning fix, I want to focus instead on eating high-fiber, high-water-content foods that also provide some of your daily requirements of nutrients. Most of my midmorning snack options are not available in vending machines, so they do require planning ahead. But this also means your snack will be in your bag when 11 a.m. rolls around, and you won't have an excuse to forgo this eating occasion.

Snack Ideas (0–100 calories):

- A piece of fruit: an apple, orange, peach, plum, banana, or pear
- Fruit salad: make your own at home or buy it anywhere; incorporate berries, melons, pineapple, grapes, kiwi, or eat these fruits on their own
- A diced mango and/or papaya
- A cup of fresh cherries
- A halved tomato seasoned with salt and pepper
- Raw red, yellow, and green pepper slices
- Carrot, celery, and cucumber sticks (try baby carrots)
- A fruit leather
- 1 cup air-popped popcorn (skip the butter and lightly sprinkle with salt and pepper)
- 8 dried apricot halves

 **CHEW ON THIS!**

"Insanity: doing the same thing over and over again and expecting different results." —Albert Einstein
Be proactive and start planning ahead for your health.

- A mini box of raisins
- 2 tablespoons of dried cherries
- 3 prunes, 3 dates, or 3 fresh or dried figs: I call these "grown-up foods" because they don't taste good until you are an adult. If you haven't tried them for a long time, trust me, they are delicious.
- A can of V8 juice or other vegetable juice (look for low-sodium versions, under 150 mg per 1-cup serving)

Savvy Girl Tip

Take care of your teeth with your midmorning snack. Go for a mini box of raisins to fight bacteria that cause dental cavities or an apple to brighten your pearly whites.

- If you absolutely crave something sweet, go for any of the 100 Calorie Packs that have become widely available. The main thing I like about these snacks is that they are preportioned and very easy to grab when you are on the go. They do, however, contain a lot of artificial stuff and high-fructose corn syrup, so limit them to once or twice a week.

Along with any of these snacks, sip on a low-cal or calorie-free drink, hot or iced:

- Go for water (sparkling or still)
- If you don't love the taste of plain water, squeeze in some lemon or lime juice. Or add fresh ginger or mint to your water bottle in the morning and take it to work.
- Try lime, orange, or raspberry-flavored sparkling water
- Save your coffee or tea until 10 a.m., after breakfast, and have it with your snack

Okay—get back to work for a couple hours . . . I'll see you for one of the highlights of every workday: lunch!

PROFILE

The Office Ennui

Deb woke up every morning dreading the coming workday. She just wasn't thrilled with her assistant position—think Pam in *The Office* without Jim to distract her—but she needed to pay the bills and wasn't getting any bites from her online resume post. Besides being completely understimulated (and in her mind, also underpaid), the problem was that her boredom led to constant opportunities for grazing. Not only would Deb dip into the candy jar on her desk throughout the day, she would routinely drop by the vending machine for a little pick-me-up when she was especially bored. Further, it was just too tempting to ignore the unhealthy food that was always sitting around the office—cookies, leftover pizza, chips, etc.—especially when Deb felt tired and grumpy (which seemed like all the time).

THE SOLUTION

When Deb contacted me, she was really down in the dumps. The first thing we decided was that she simply could not allow herself to eat the food lying around her office. It was way too hard for her to control herself once she got started nibbling. We figured out that the best way for her to combat these temptations was to plan ahead to ensure healthy alternatives were always within arm's reach. On Monday, I advised Deb to bring in a bag of fruit for the week. Deb liked this option and told me that she keeps a "please don't touch if your name is not Deb" sign on the bag so she can put it in the office kitchen. Additionally, we agreed that Deb should keep healthy snacks in her desk drawer—think high-fiber cereal, cans of soup, dried fruit, and low-calorie granola bars. Deb also invested in a nice selection of teas. When she feels like consuming but isn't actually hungry, a steaming hot zero-calorie drink proved to be a great distraction. Lastly, Deb got rid of the candy jar on her desk—there was no reason to have sweet treats tempting her all day long.

PART 3

Noontime

CHAPTER 8

Think Outside the Lunch Box

WHEN IT COMES to our midday meal, many of us choose whatever is most convenient or perhaps forgo lunch altogether as a tactic to save calories, time, or money. Others build up a ravenous appetite (often because they have skipped breakfast and/or their midmorning snack), watching the clock for an opportunity to jump fork-first into a midday calorie trap. And for others, lunch just means more work—a catered business meeting or taking a client out. In this chapter, I will show you how to seize the opportunity of your midday meal to instill Healthy Habit #4: Eat a lunch containing high-fiber and high-water-content foods, as well as a portion of lean protein. **Aim for 400 to 600 calories.** Whether you are eating out or brown-bagging it, lunch is an important meal for every woman and can be an excellent time to get in some of your 5 A Day fruit and veggie requirement via typical entrees such as salad, sandwiches, and soup.

A Word about Cheese

Before we move on to these lunch meals, I want to take a quick moment to delve into cheese because I know it is a daily fix for many of us—often starting at lunchtime as a prominent player in salads and sandwiches or enjoyed with crackers as an afternoon treat. Cheese can be a healthy part of your diet if you limit whole-milk cheeses to special occasions and regularly enjoy reduced-fat or fat-free options in portion-controlled amounts. **Go for about 1 ounce**, which is the size of four dice. Generally treat cheese like a condiment—to flavor and enhance your food—rather than as the key ingredient. For instance, instead of a blue cheese salad, which often features up to 4 ounces of cheese, go for a grilled chicken breast salad that is lightly sprinkled with parmesan. If you are dining out and order the warm goat cheese salad, for example, ask your server how that "warm" cheese is prepared—you may be surprised to find it is often *fried*. Here are some good everyday parameters for cheese:

◆ Sprinkle salads with crumbled goat or feta cheese—they are naturally lower in fat and calories than most cow's milk cheeses. Or, try parmesan—a small amount packs in a lot of flavor . . . delicious! (Hint: Use a lemon zester to grate hard cheeses—you will net a finer grate with less cheese but it will be more evenly distributed).

◆ For sandwiches, try Alpine Lace cheeses—they are sold at deli counters and are low-fat—go for the reduced-fat deli Swiss cheese. Or try sharp cheeses, like cheddar, which allow you to enjoy a punch of flavor in a small portion. Ask for one slice only (which is about an ounce) or try a couple slices of Cabot 50% Reduced Fat Sharp Cheddar, which is delicious and a little friendlier to your waistline.

◆ For snacks, go for low-fat mozzarella or reduced-fat string cheese—try Polly-O Part Skim Mozzarella. Or try a spreadable cheese like Laughing Cow Light on whole wheat crackers or with veggies.

◆ When cooking, use low-fat ricotta or cottage cheese for lasagna or casseroles.

◆ Save soft cheeses like Brie and Camembert for special occasions (I love a great cheese and fruit plate as much as anyone, but only now and then).

As an aside, most lactose-intolerant people will have little or no trouble eating ripened or aged cheeses. This is because these cheeses are treated with enzymes and bacteria that break down lactose over time and form lactic acid instead, which will not cause distress. The longer a cheese is aged, the less lactose it will contain. Some commonly aged cheeses include: parmesan, Romano, Asiago, some cheddars, and Gruyère.

Okay—back to the three staples that characterize lunch:

#1: Lean on Salads

Most of us know that not all salads are created equal. In fact, the calorie content ranges drastically—literally anywhere from 50 to upwards of 2,000 calories per salad, depending on your fixings and dressing. Eating the right salads every day is a fabulous way to fill up on the best foods—veggies and lean protein—and to fulfill your 5 A Day goal. And here's an added bonus: Research has indicated that women who eat two servings of vegetables per day tend to look younger than their non-veggie-eating peers. Think how many years you can shave off if you start getting your veggies *now*. Whether you make your lunchtime salad at home and bring it to work, pick up a premade salad at the local deli or sandwich shop, or take a midday trip to the make-your-own salad spot, here are some strategies for building a healthy, delicious, and satiating meal without breaking your calorie budget.

Healthy Salad Building Blocks

◆ **Lettuce:** Try spinach, romaine (a.k.a. Cos), arugula (a.k.a. rocket), Bibb (a.k.a. Boston or butter), mesculin, and iceberg. These make up the base of every salad; all are exceptionally low in calories, over 90 percent water, and help fill us up. Typically the darker the lettuce, the more nutrients, specifically vitamin C, folate, beta carotene, vitamin K, and potassium. Iceberg is the least nutritious and should be used with other salad greens for crunch, not as the only type of lettuce you eat. Branch out if you haven't already.

◆ **Nonstarchy veggies:** Aim for ingredients like beets, carrots, mushrooms, celery, onions, cucumber, tomatoes, asparagus, broccoli, peppers, artichoke hearts, hearts of palm, fennel, and fresh herbs. These are virtually calorie-free and filled with vitamins and minerals. Try to choose three to four of these goodies to get enough variety without overaccessorizing.

◆ **Protein:** It's important to add some protein to your salad so you stay satiated all afternoon. Some good options include grilled, roasted, or baked chicken or turkey breast; shrimp; salmon or tuna (canned or fresh, no mayo); or tofu. A serving size of lean protein is about 3 ounces, or the size of a deck of cards.

◆ **Fiber:** Beans are a great source of fiber and protein. Look for salads that feature beans as a main ingredient, or add about ½ cup as a fixing to your own salad. Some good options to try include black beans, chickpeas, white beans, lima beans, pinto beans, green beans, or kidney beans.

◆ **Healthy fat:** Aim to add 1 to 2 tablespoons of an unsaturated, heart-healthy fat to your salad. Try avocado, nuts (pecans, walnuts, pine nuts), seeds (toasted sesame or sunflower), or olives (green or black in oil). These will add flavor and richness to your meal; just be sure to stick to this small portion as these foods are high in calories and can easily be overeaten.

◆ **Fruit:** Some salads are savory while others are a little sweet. If you like the latter, toss in ½ cup of fresh fruit—try oranges, apples, or pears. A tablespoon-sized sprinkling of dried fruit will also do the trick—try figs, cherries, or cranberries.

Beware of the potential to fall victim to overaccessorizing at salad bars and make-your-own salad shops. Less is more (and usually cheaper too). Below, I've listed some things to skip when creating a salad or buying one preprepared. A hint: If the salad you are about to order sounds naughty, it probably is. Skip the fried chicken salad, and in general, avoid these extras:

◆ **Cheese:** Skip it altogether or try sprinkling in less than 1 ounce of cheese to flavor your salad. If your salad comes with more cheese than you expected, don't feel guilty about taking off the excess—this is good plate waste.

◆ **Crunchies:** As a rule, skip the croutons, Chinese noodles, fried onions, tortilla chips, and bacon bits altogether on a daily basis.

◆ **Fried protein:** Skip the chicken or fish if it is breaded, crunchy, crispy, or fried.

And now, for the finishing touch. A salad just isn't a salad without a little bit of dressing. Below are some healthy options. For each recommendation, try to stick to a 2- to 4-tablespoon serving, maximum. And order your salad dressing on the side, *dip your fork into it, and then spear your food*—you will get the most flavor for the least calories.

Savvy Girl Tip

Do not feel like you need to clean your plate. With our out-of-control portion sizes and overproduction of empty calories, leaving some "plate waste," or excess food, on your plate is imperative. Either take leftovers home for another meal or just toss them. You should feel guiltier about putting plate waste in your body than in the trash.

◆ **Healthy oils:** Go for dressings made with olive or canola oil. The unsaturated fat in these heart-healthy oils will help you absorb the fat-soluble vitamins (specifically beta carotene and vitamin K) from your veggies. Without it, your salad is *less* beneficial to your health. So, actually, it is best to avoid fat-free vinaigrettes and enjoy a little of the right type of fat without guilt.

◆ **Healthy acids:** Salad dressing is typically made from oil (above) and an acid—either vinegar, lemon, or lime juice. These acids add flavor to your veggies without any calories.

◆ **Creamy dressing:** Stay away from thick, "mayonnaisey" salad dressings that are full of saturated fat. These have no place in your everyday salad repertoire. Sorry, blue cheese, ranch, Russian, and Caesar, you're for special occasions only (like once or twice a month).

◆ **My standard, everyday salad dressing:** Whisk together 2 parts red wine vinegar with 1 part olive oil, a squeeze of lemon juice, and a sprinkling of *sugar* and pepper. This yummy dressing adds flavor to salad without overpowering the taste of the vegetables.

Some flavors just taste better together. When you're faced with such a plethora of ingredients, it's easy to create a monster in a bowl. Here are my suggestions for salad combinations that fall within your 400- to 600-calorie budget. Make these at home or at the salad bar—they are healthy *and* delicious—and top them with a heart-healthy vinaigrette:

◆ **The Autumn:** Spinach, artichoke hearts, goat cheese, pecans, and dried cranberries

◆ **The Mexican:** Romaine, tomato, salsa, black beans, avocado, and cheddar cheese

◆ **The "Fresh":** Arugula, beets, carrots, tuna (water packed, no mayo), and chickpeas

- **The Vegetarian:** Bibb lettuce, tomatoes, mushrooms, onions, sunflower seeds, and tofu (or grilled fish)

- **The Greek:** Mesculin, tomatoes, cucumber, olives, red onion, feta cheese, and grilled chicken

- **The Modified Cobb:** Iceberg and arugula, tomatoes, avocado, hard-boiled egg white, grilled chicken breast, and turkey bacon

#2: The Dish on the Sandwich

Nothing satisfies like a sandwich when you are craving some carbs to go with your veggies and protein. As with salads, the calorie content of sandwiches ranges dramatically—depending on the bread, fixings, and condiments. Whether you're picking up from a deli counter, making it at home, or ordering at a restaurant, here's how to build a healthy and satisfying sandwich that will add to your 5 A Day goal and fit into your calorie budget:

Healthy Sandwich Building Blocks

- **Bread:** What's a sandwich without the bread? Choose whole grain or whole wheat sliced bread, and toast it to bring out the nutty flavor and crunch. Also, you can always try a 4- or 6-inch whole wheat pita, but skip the extra-large 9-inch varieties—they get very caloric. Skip options like Italian, sourdough, or white breads on a daily basis. Those Kaiser rolls and baguettes look yummy but are often loaded with empty calories, *at least* 50 more per sandwich, and usually without much in the way of fiber. Generally, avoid wraps at all costs—a typical wrap alone packs 300+ calories—approximately 100 calories more than a couple slices of bread or a pita.

- **Protein:** When it comes to deli meats, choose lean and extra-lean varieties—either called "95% fat free" or "with only 5% fat"; go for roasted or smoked turkey or ham. Other great options include plain water-packed tuna (no mayo), grilled chicken breast, or poached or grilled salmon.

- Veggie burgers, a common lunchtime protein, range widely in healthfulness, as some contain a lot of sodium, oil, and cheese. The main ingredients you should look for are vegetables, grains (brown rice, oats, and barley), nuts, textured vegetable protein (TVP), and legumes (beans, lentils). The good thing is most patties are relatively small and typically contain no more than 175 calories.

- **Cheese:** It's hard to imagine a sandwich without the cheese, but I'll bet you will be surprised how little you will miss it if you exclude it from your daily sandwich. If you aren't ready to go that far, make sure to order your sandwich with only one slice of cheese and/or go for the reduced-fat options. Further, always choose *either* cheese *or* another fat like mayo or avocado. One of these is enough to add richness to your sandwich.

- **Veggies:** Whenever possible, try to load your sandwich with vegetables—the standard lettuce, tomato, pickle, and onion are great, but also look for ingredients like cucumber, fresh red or green peppers, spinach, or sprouts.

  - Beware of veggie sandwiches posing as healthy but containing roasted or grilled veggies dripping in oil or paired with copious amounts of cheese. These are inferior choices to lean meat alternatives or fresh vegetable sandwiches.

- **Condiments:** If you like a little extra kick to your sandwich, use brown or yellow mustard, salsa, hummus, chutneys, vinegar, pepper, and herbs such as oregano or basil. Stay away from high-calorie and high-fat options such as mayo, tapenade, pesto, "spreads," and anything with the

Save yourself hundreds of calories by choosing the healthier version of your favorite sandwich.		
2 slices of whole wheat bread, 4 ounces sliced turkey, mustard, & unlimited veggies (~300 calories)	*vs*	2 slices of white bread, 4 ounces sliced turkey, 1 tablespoon mayo, 2 slices cheddar cheese (~625 calories)
2 slices of whole wheat bread, 4 ounces plain tuna, mustard, & unlimited veggies (~300 calories)	*vs*	2 slices of white bread, 4 ounces tuna salad with 2 tablespoons mayo, 1 slice cheddar cheese (~615 calories)
2 ounces avocado on 2 slices whole wheat toast (~250 calories, ~1.2 grams saturated fat)	*vs*	grilled cheese sandwich on white bread with 2 ounces cheddar cheese (~400 calories, ~12 grams saturated fat)

word "aioli," which is basically a fancy word for flavored mayonnaise.

The benefit of making a sandwich at home is that you have complete control over all the ingredients. Here are some of my favorite sandwich combinations when I'm brown-bagging it:

◆ **Variation on a classic:** I love fresh, all-natural peanut or almond butter (try grinding your own at health stores or in select Whole Foods). Go for 2 tablespoons of nut butter with 2 teaspoons of your favorite jam or jelly. (Note: Jam is made from whole fruit while jelly is made from fruit juice.) Or better yet, top a peanut butter sandwich with any fresh fruit, like thinly sliced banana, apples, or strawberries.

- **California Special:** Spread one-fourth of an avocado on a piece of whole-wheat toast, and add a pinch of salt and pepper. If you want a kick, sprinkle on some crushed red pepper or a squirt of lemon or lime juice and enjoy.
- **Vegetarian Sandwich:** Use hummus as your protein and fill the sandwich with fresh veggies you love. Alternatively, if you're stuck on cheese, use low-fat mozzarella as your protein and add fresh tomatoes and basil (or any other veggies you like). Toast your sandwich so it is warm and even more appealing.

Give me a side of . . .

A lunch built around a sandwich somehow does not feel complete without a "side." Chips have played life partner to the sandwich for ages, but here I must advocate divorce. Chips are to eating what smoking is to breathing—a quick fix that, if allowed to become a habit, will clog your arteries for a lifetime. If you must, eat a serving of chips on the weekend, but definitely cut them out of your daily habit, even if they are "baked" or reduced-fat. Here are some ideas for healthy, satisfying sides:

- **Pickles:** Most sandwich shops and delis give them to you for free. Eat your pickle. It is low in calories and packed with flavor.
- **Crudités:** Try a handful of crunchy baby carrots or celery, cucumber, or red pepper sticks. Dip them in hummus or vinaigrette for extra flavor.
- **Salad:** Many restaurants will allow you to replace chips or fries with a small side salad, and small, prepackaged salads are often available in refrigerated cases at sandwich shops.
- **Soup:** A small cup of a broth-based soup will help fill you up without adding a lot of extra calories.

- **Seaweed salad:** Always available at a Japanese or sushi joint, but increasingly available even at the grocery store.

- **Fresh fruit or fruit salad:** Again, toss an apple or pear into your bag the night before, or grab a small, premade fruit salad at the same place you get your sandwich.

- **Yogurt or cottage cheese:** A cup of either is filling and will give you a nice dose of calcium—30 percent of your daily requirement.

#3: The Skinny on Soup

Soup can play partner to your salad and sandwich options, or it can provide a great midday meal in and of itself—*if* you choose a healthy soup. Broth-based soups are generally very low in calories. In fact, 1 cup is usually only about 100 calories, due to its naturally high water content. As a result, you can eat a large serving of soup and feel full without consuming a ton of calories. Many soups are also naturally low in fat, saturated fat, and cholesterol, and they are often full of a variety of antioxidant-rich vegetables to add to your 5 A Day goal. In addition, soup is difficult to eat quickly, so you are forced to take some time to savor it. Whether you eat soup as an appetizer, side, or main course, just make sure to follow the basics. For the most nutrition in your bowl, aim for:

- Chicken or vegetable broth–based soups
- Bean-based soups such as black bean, split pea, lentil, or minestrone with beans
- Tomato-based soups such as tomato, vegetable, Manhattan clam chowder, gazpacho, or vegetarian or turkey chili

  Avoid soups that are:

- Cream-based and thus packed with saturated fat: cream of mushroom, corn chowder, or New England clam chowder

◆ Full of sodium: Read labels if available and do not salt your soup before tasting it. Order a small cup to control your sodium intake, especially if you have high blood pressure.

In the same time as it takes you to go out and get your lunch each day, you can make a simple and delicious batch of soup that you'll have on hand all week long. These are my recipes and they are easy for anyone to make. Although each recipe has only a few ingredients, these soups are full of nutrition.

◆ **Black Bean Soup:** In a blender, combine 2 cups or 1 can of low-sodium chicken or vegetable broth and two 15-ounce cans of drained black beans. Blend, transfer to a large pot, and cook over high heat until the soup boils. Season as desired. I recommend salt, pepper, and fresh cilantro, and if you want to go all-out, sauté half of an onion, chopped, on the side and either blend it in or sprinkle it on top. If you are eating this at home, you can also add a tablespoon of freshly grated sharp cheddar.

◆ **Winter Squash or Carrot Soup:** In a blender, combine 2 cups or 1 can of chicken or vegetable broth and 3 cups of steamed winter squash or carrots. Blend, transfer to a large pot, and cook over high heat until the soup boils. Season as desired. I recommend a pinch of salt, pepper, and either a pinch of sage, a pinch of cinnamon, or 1 tablespoon of grated fresh ginger.

◆ **Low-fat Cream of Broccoli or Asparagus Soup:** In a blender, combine 2 cups or 1 can of chicken or vegetable broth and 3 cups of steamed broccoli or asparagus. Add ½ cup of low-fat milk. Blend, transfer to a large pot, and cook over medium heat until soup boils. Season as desired. I recommend just a pinch of salt and pepper. If you are eating this at home, sprinkle with 1 tablespoon of freshly grated parmesan cheese.

◆ **Minestrone Soup**—Combine 4 cups vegetable broth, 4 cups water, 4 chopped carrots, 4 chopped celery stalks, 1 chopped yellow onion, and 3 cloves of minced garlic in a large pot and simmer on medium-high heat for 40 minutes, covered. Then add 1 can of drained kidney beans, 1 can of drained chickpeas, 1½ cups of uncooked whole wheat pasta (try bowties), and a 12-ounce can of diced tomatoes. Cook uncovered for another 25 minutes on high heat, and season to taste.

If soup alone doesn't quite satisfy you, try combining your soup entrée with a little something extra. The soup meals below are all 500 calories or less:

◆ 2 cups of black bean soup and a large green salad

◆ 2 cups of chicken vegetable soup, half a tuna sandwich, and a handful of baby carrots

◆ 2 cups of tomato soup with 4 ounces of grilled salmon or chicken and a piece of fruit

◆ 2 cups of minestrone soup with a small whole wheat seedy roll, 1 tablespoon of peanut butter, and a piece of fruit

◆ 2 cups of winter squash soup with a small low-fat Caesar salad

◆ 2 cups of vegetarian chili over ½ cup brown rice, sprinkled with 1 tablespoon of low-fat cheddar cheese and a piece of fruit

◆ 2 cups of lentil soup, 6 saltine crackers, and a cup of low-fat yogurt

◆ 2 cups of miso soup and 1 California sushi roll

◆ 1 cup of low-fat cream of broccoli soup with ½ toasted whole wheat bagel, 1 tablespoon of light cream cheese, and tomato slices

Lunch Meeting Woes

Whether you are stuck in a conference room for your midday meal or a sales rep is providing it for your office, most catered office lunches tend to be calorie traps, and they can feel hard to avoid since the food is right under your nose. But don't despair: There are ways to navigate the lunch meeting spread. Frequent offerings at such meetings include sandwiches, pasta salads, chips, fruit, cookies, sodas, and bottled water. If you normally go for something like a tuna salad sandwich, chips, a can of soda, and a couple of cookies, here are some strategies for choosing a healthier working lunch that will save you from packing on unwanted pounds.

◆ **Beverage:** It's a no-brainer to always skip the full-calorie soda and go for a bottle of water (or a diet soda, if you must—but again, a maximum of two per day). If you simply switch from drinking a 12-ounce can of soda five days a week to drinking water or diet soda instead, you can save yourself up to 10 pounds per year. What's more, there are *10 teaspoons of sugar in one can of regular soda*—measure that out into a clear glass and you will be horrified.

◆ **Premade sandwiches:** Peel away excess cheese—a standard slice (about 1 ounce) of cheese is roughly 100 calories. Over the course of a year, skipping just one slice five days a week saves you approximately 26,000 calories, or 7½ pounds. Go for the lunch meat over the mayo-based chicken or tuna salad; you'll save more than 100 calories per sandwich, or another 7½ pounds over the course of a year.

◆ **Condiments:** If those convenient little packets tempt you, go for the mustard instead of the mayonnaise. One tablespoon of mayo has about 100 calories, whereas 1 table-spoon of mustard only adds about 15 calories to your meal. By making this adjustment each day, five days a week, you save yourself up to 22,100 calories and about 6 pounds per year.

◆ **Sides:** Skip the chips and the pasta salad and go for the fruit. A serving of chips—1 ounce or about 20 chips—is about 150 calories, whereas a serving of fruit is more like 75 calories. Plus, you get to check off one more serving toward your 5 A Day goal. Make this switch every day during the workweek and save yourself approximately 19,500 calories or 5½ pounds per year. If you forgo the pasta salad for the fruit, you will be saving 125 calories per day (½ cup of the oily stuff runs you in the neighborhood of 200 calories) and 32,500 calories, or about 9 pounds per year.

◆ **Dessert:** If you're really craving something sweet after the fruit, share a cookie with your colleague. The chocolate chip cookies offered on most catering trays will cost you another 300 calories. Halve that five days a week and save up to 39,000 calories, or 11 pounds, over the course of a year.

◆ **The biggest rule: If you don't love it, don't eat it.** Don't waste your calories on food that doesn't satisfy you. You can always eat after the meeting or brown-bag it if you know about the lunch meeting in advance. Sure, people may look at you funny, but trust me, they will be looks of envy when they see your meal compared to theirs.

Desk drawer staples

Cans or microwaveable bowls of soup and individual serving packets of whole wheat crackers can come in handy on a rainy day when you don't feel like heading outside on your lunch break.

◆ **Think outside the box.** If it makes sense in your office environment, make your monthly office lunch meeting a healthy potluck and bring something delicious and nutritious. Or, if possible, make your client meeting an afternoon walk outside instead of a lunch meeting . . . you are not supposed to work through meals anyway. They should be breaks in your day.

Fast Food . . . to Your Hips

We Americans get (and deserve) a lot of criticism for our fast food habit—but let's face it: Low prices and convenience are attractive. Given our schedules, I cannot realistically tell you *never* to eat fast food and expect you always to plan ahead, shop at Whole Foods, and cook at home. Therefore, I would like to help you choose a chain where your odds of successful eating are high when you walk in the door. And it goes without saying: The most popular fast food items—a burger, french fries, or fried chicken—have no place in your daily diet.

At some of our country's largest chains—McDonald's, Burger King, KFC, and Jack in the Box—choose the lesser evil. The best option at these establishments is usually a grilled chicken sandwich—hold the bacon, mayo, and cheese—or a grilled chicken salad with the light vinaigrette. True, the small hamburgers at these joints are sometimes less caloric than these options, but they usually contain more preservatives. You can also try a kid's meal to cut your portions down—these typically come with healthy side options like fruit and yogurt. When it comes to pizza chains, Domino's, Pizza Hut, and Papa John's are never more than a delivery boy away. Always choose thin crust pizza, load it with veggies, hold the meat, and share it with your colleagues. Again, I strongly recommend that these chains not be part of your workday routine.

Fast Food Joints

Below I've listed a few fast food joints that aren't so bad if you order carefully. Here are my suggestions for safe menu picks:

◆ **Wendy's:** Go for the chili (hold the cheese and sour cream), salad bar (use our salad tips on page 82), or grilled chicken sandwich.

◆ **Subway:** Order a 6-inch sub on a whole wheat roll and load it up with fresh veggies. Substitute oil and vinegar for mayo and skip the cheese, as it is rather bland and I guarantee you won't miss it.

◆ **Quizno's:** Stick with a small or regular-size sandwich on a whole wheat roll. Given that their sandwiches are often constructed around a sauce and/or melted cheese, chose one or the other and always skip the mayo.

◆ **Boston Market:** Try the rotisserie chicken (without the skin) and a side of chicken soup, fresh steamed veggies, a small salad, or a fresh fruit salad.

◆ **Baja Fresh:** Create your own burrito and preferably go Bare Style (skip the tortilla and have your burrito in a bowl). Pile on fresh salsa, beans, charbroiled chicken, grilled veggies, fresh onions,

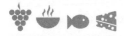 CHEW ON THIS!

McDonald's has a budget of $1 billion to advertise their food while the government has $1 million to advertise the 5 A Day fruits and vegetables initiative.[2] Use your DVR to fast-forward through the fast food commercials and put the documentary film Super Size Me *at the top of your Netflix queue.*

and cilantro; skip the sour cream and rice, go easy on the cheese, and enjoy a little of the fresh guacamole or avocado.

◆ **Au Bon Pain:** Look for the broth- and bean-based soups and opt for the whole grain bread over the crackers. Go for the prepackaged salads, but pick off excess cheese and croutons and chose a vinaigrette dressing. Order a build-your-own sandwich using the tips discussed on page 85.

Okay—lunch is over. Nice work, ladies—you're halfway home. . . .

PROFILE

Fast Food Next Exit

Leslie is a pharmaceutical sales rep living in Los Angeles. She made a good living and enjoyed her career—it was social and different every day, and she knew she could never stand the monotony of a typical desk job. However, Leslie often felt prisoner to her car (and the traffic on the 405). In a hurry to get from one doctor to the next, Leslie often ended up stopping at the first fast food drive-thru she saw to grab a quick lunch and, let's face it, salad was impossible to eat while she was driving. Further, Leslie typically guzzled coffee throughout the day instead of snacking on something more nutritious because it gave her a quick boost of energy and did not require any planning ahead. Her favorite was the 20-ounce Mocha Latte with soy milk from Coffee Bean and Tea Leaf (she usually had at least two a day). Leslie had put on 10 pounds and found me on the Internet, desperate for some advice.

THE SOLUTION

Clearly, lunch was a big problem for Leslie, so we decided to tackle this first. We discussed the fast food joints that she should avoid altogether and those where her odds of successful eating were highest. We went over menus to pick out meals that would fit in with her fast-paced life and calorie budget—a Subway 6-inch veggie sandwich or a Wendy's grilled chicken sandwich. I recommended that she program her car's GPS system to automatically find only the chains we deemed good options along her route, so she wouldn't just stop at the first brightly colored sign that caught her eye.

As for her coffee habit, just one of her coffee drinks was almost 500 calories and provided little nutrition. Because Leslie was always in her car, I advised that she keep a cooler in her trunk stocked with bottled water, seltzer, and fruit. Further, along with her favorite hand lotion and lip balm, she could also stash sugar-free mint chewing gum in her glove compartment, which would help her to stay satiated and keep her breath fresh for the doctors.

Finally, Leslie and I discussed proactive ways to combat her boredom while stuck in traffic. She was already listening to NPR and chatting with friends via her Bluetooth, but I suggested trying to learn a new language on a CD or downloading the audio version of her favorite book or magazine onto her iPod.

Leslie e-mailed me with great news: She has lost 11 pounds—so she actually weighs less than ever before. But the main thing that she cannot get over is how much more energy she has all day long. She attributes this to both her healthier lunch (she no longer has a food coma after eating), along with staying well-hydrated and forgoing caffeine as her only source of energy. Plus, her car time is less painful now that she is listening to *The Economist*'s audio edition.

CHAPTER 9

The Afternoon Slump

SO YOU'VE EATEN a healthy lunch, but as you finish the last bite, you begin to crave something sweet. This is the perfect time to implement Healthy Habit #5: If you have a sweet tooth, and most of us women do, have a "sweet nothing" every day. As your nutritionist, I feel that dessert is such an important part of the day that we should make it a habit—but a low-calorie one. Sweet nothings are your **every-single-day 0- to 150-calorie dessert "do's."** I have found that women who allow themselves a sweet indulgence every day do not have cravings that lead to outrageous binges and don't feel deprived. Here are some desserts that are okay to eat habitually, after lunch or at any time during the day. Partake in the sweet life without sacrificing your figure or your health!

Steamy, Sweet Drinks

◆ A decaf skim cappuccino sprinkled with cinnamon and a small, plain biscotti

◆ Hot chocolate: Try the Nestlé or Swiss Miss 25- to 35-calorie packets mixed with hot water

- Homemade ginger tea: combine grated fresh ginger, lemon juice, and 1 teaspoon of honey in a mug and pour in hot water; this is an excellent after-lunch drink, as the ginger aids digestion
- Orange, mint, or chai tea, which are all naturally infused with sweetness

No-Guilt Confections

- 1 ounce dark chocolate: You have probably heard the hype, but this dessert really *is* full of antioxidants, and even small amounts taste decadent and rich. In addition, dark chocolate has less sugar than milk chocolate, and most of the saturated fat in dark chocolate comes from stearic acid, which converts in your body to heart-healthy oleic acid (also found in olive oil). Dark chocolate has even been proven to reduce high blood pressure.
- A mini-sized peppermint patty
- Hard sucking candies: If you feel you can handle the risk that comes with having a bag of candies around, try 1 to 3 per day (Jolly Ranchers, butterscotch, LifeSavers, etc.) or just go for a lollipop
- A Viactiv calcium chew: They come in chocolate, caramel, and raspberry flavors and can be found in the supplement/vitamin section of the grocery and drugstore.
- A single-serving cup of sugar-free Jell-O or pudding, any flavor

"Dressed-Up" Fruit

- Frozen grapes or fresh Concord grapes, which are particularly sweet and juicy (a serving is about 15 grapes)
- A frozen banana
- A pomegranate (peel it in a bowl filled with water to separate seeds from the rind and enjoy)

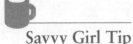

Savvy Girl Tip

To increase the size of your Sweet Nothing, add ½ cup of skim milk to your ½ cup serving of low-fat ice cream or frozen yogurt. Delicious and you get extra calcium!

- Fresh berries with a touch of balsamic vinegar and fat-free Cool Whip or Reddi-Wip.

- A cup of fresh cherries

- A cup of mango, papaya, pineapple, or watermelon chunks

- A whole peeled kiwi

- A peach diced into ½ cup of nonfat vanilla yogurt

- A baked apple (halve it and bake at 350°F for 45 to 60 minutes), sprinkled with cinnamon and topped with a tablespoon of nonfat sour cream

- A baked pear (halve it and bake at 350°F for 25 minutes), sprinkled with cinnamon and topped with a tablespoon of nonfat vanilla yogurt

Frozen Treats

An ice cream craving may actually be a sign of thirst—try cold water before you indulge to make sure you really want a dessert.

- Try preportioned ice cream treats like Skinny Cow ice cream sandwiches, Tofutti Cuties (these are nondairy), Fudgsicles, or 100-percent-fruit frozen pops (I like Dreyer's/Edy's lemon, lime, or strawberry)

- Portion out ½ cup of low-fat ice cream, frozen yogurt, or sorbet

Snack Time, Take 2

With a yawn, you glance at the clock. It's 3:30 p.m. and, as usual, you are feeling lethargic and in need of a pick-me-up to get you through the remainder of the workday. Time to remind you of Healthy Habit #3: Aim for a midmorning and a midafternoon snack every day, in addition to your three regular meals. Let's discuss **your more substantial daily snack (100 to 200 calories)**. If find that most of my clients get very sluggish in the afternoon, and many do not eat dinner until 8 p.m. or later. The afternoon is an ideal time to fuel up to keep your metabolism going. A carefully planned snack can boost your energy and save you calories later. Plus, you will not be starving going into dinner, so you will be less likely to overeat—I promise. Instead of rushing to the nearest bakery or coffee shop for a decadent or caffeinated fix, I will show you how to choose the right kind of snack that will satisfy and help you meet your daily nutritional needs—especially your calcium requirement.

Here are some great high-calcium options to ward off the afternoon doldrums. They are all in the 100- to 200-calorie range:

◆ 1 cup of nonfat or low-fat yogurt (toss in 1 tablespoon of low-fat granola or fresh fruit)

◆ 1½ cups of low-fat cottage cheese paired with fruit (try a peach, a plum, or a cup of fresh berries) or veggies (try a cup of diced tomatoes or cucumbers)

◆ 1 ounce of cheese (4 dice-sized cubes or 1 slice); pair with a piece of fruit or about 6 whole grain crackers like low-fat Triscuits, Wheat Thins, or Wasa crackers

◆ ½ cup of edamame (shelled soybeans); buy a bag of these frozen, boiled soybeans, and pack a handful in the a.m.—they will be thawed and ready to eat by snack time

◆ 1 ounce nuts, such as almonds, walnuts, pecans, or cashews

◆ 6 ounces of nonfat frozen yogurt

◆ 1 cup nonfat or low-fat milk or calcium-fortified soy milk paired with 1 Hershey's miniature Special Dark chocolate or a small square of any high-quality 70 percent cocoa dark chocolate

◆ 1 serving size of high-fiber cereal in 1 cup of skim milk

Here are some other tasty and nutritious afternoon snack ideas in the 100- to 200-calorie range:

◆ An apple or banana with 1 tablespoon of peanut or almond butter

◆ Veggies or about 6 whole wheat crackers with 3 tablespoons of hummus or black bean dip; grab an extra salad dressing container when you are picking up a salad and use for hummus (or any other condiment you prefer, like peanut butter or salsa)

◆ Homemade trail mix—add 1 tablespoon almonds, 1 tablespoon dried cherries, 1 tablespoon dark chocolate chips, and 1 tablespoon Fiber One cereal. This is about 200 calories and delicious.

◆ 1 sliced, hard-boiled egg with about 6 crackers or 1 piece of toast

◆ 1 cup of broth-based soup

◆ 1 cup baked tortilla chips with 1 tablespoon of guacamole and 3 tablespoons salsa

 CHEW ON THIS!

In females, 99 percent of total body mineral content is achieved by 22 years of age (i.e., your opportunity to build new bone peaks).[1] From then on, only lifestyle choices can delay your rate of bone loss. Make sure to eat calcium-rich foods through the day and try weight-bearing exercises at the gym to increase bone strength and density.

- An energy bar that is high in calcium, fiber, and protein—I recommend Luna bars, LaraBars, Balance 100 calorie bars, and Gnu Flavor & Fiber bars
- A granola bar that has more than 3 grams of fiber—I recommend Trader Joe's Sweet and Savory granola bars, Nature's Valley Granola Bars, and Kashi TLC Chewy Trail Mix bars

Victim of the vending machine? Typically I like to avoid these snack dispensers altogether, but when you're in a pinch, try one of these options over the candy bar or bag of sugar cookies:

- Honey whole wheat pretzels
- Soy chips
- Nature's Valley Granola Bars
- Individual package of Fig Newtons
- Animal crackers
- Cracker Jack
- SnackWells 4-pack cookies

If you still feel tired after your afternoon snack, here are some tips for gaining that last push of momentum to get you through the workday:

- Leave your desk and get some air, stretch, and even burn a few calories by walking around the block. Moving around will get your blood pumping and increase your oxygen levels, giving you an instant boost.

- Give yourself a mini massage—go for some of our most sensitive pressure points: your temples, jaw, and shoulders.

- Tune up with iTunes—a great way out of a slump is to throw on your earbuds and listen to a playlist that pumps you up.

Desk drawer staples

It's always good to have Luna Bars, granola bars, and low-cal hot cocoa packets on hand for an easy afternoon snack or pre-gym energy boost.

- Think mint—try peppermint tea, gum, or mints; it can actually signal your brain to become more alert.

- Drink water—the oxygen component will give you energy without calories or chemicals. As a matter of fact, your fatigue may even result from being mildly dehydrated. When you are lethargic, ask yourself: "Have I had enough water today?"

It's finally 5:00 (or for some of you, 6:00 or 7:00). Onward and upward to the best part of every working day—getting out of the office. If you've made good choices throughout your day, you won't be ravenous on your way home from work and feel tempted to dropkick the person who stole your seat on the subway. Now is your time to relax for a few precious hours, so don't waste it!

PROFILE

Food, Summa Cum Laude

Becca graduated from a prestigious hotel school and became a catering manager. She was the ultimate foodie, which made her excellent at her job. She loved wine and bread and cheese and soups and stocks and sauces galore, but above all else, she loved her sweets. The hazards of her job were clear: It was extremely hard to work around food all day and not overeat. Moreover, sharing her workspace with a pastry chef was hard on her figure. By 4 p.m. every day, simple cravings turned into serious calorie bombs. Becca would leave work riddled with guilt and upset by her inability to control herself.

THE SOLUTION

Becca needed to learn how to satisfy her sweet tooth while practicing some restraint. Together we came up with a list of Sweet Nothings that Becca could eat every day without guilt. Because Becca was a chocoholic, a low-calorie hot cocoa with a few mini marshmallows or 1 ounce of 70 percent dark chocolate after lunch would do the trick. Becca still indulges in the treats whipped up by the pastry chef every now and then, but on a daily basis, she has found better ways to curb her sweet tooth.

PART 4

Evening

CHAPTER 10

Happy Hour—
Cocktails, Anyone?

MOST OF US hardly need an excuse to order a cocktail at the end of a long workday. You've heard the hype about red wine being beneficial to your health, but you're likely also aware of the ill effects of alcohol. So what is the deal? Is it healthy to indulge in a daily drink? And what is the difference between drinking one alcoholic beverage a day versus drinking four or five at one sitting a couple times a week? Because drinking is not for every woman, I would like to introduce Healthy Habit #6 as our first *optional* habit: per the Dietary Guidelines for women, drink up to one alcoholic beverage per day.[1] I will lay out the facts about alcohol and women in this chapter so you can decide for yourself how to handle your booze. I will also provide nutritional strategies to alleviate the worst hangovers and tips on how to reduce and quit one of the nastiest fixes that sometimes accompanies drinking: smoking cigarettes.

Calorie Control

The recommendation for women who are *not* pregnant is to drink up to one alcoholic beverage per day. This is based on years of research that indicates that risk of disease, including certain cancers, increases when we consume more than this. The chart opposite provides the recommended serving sizes, approximate calorie levels, and percent alcohol content for some of our most common happy hour elixirs.

As you can see, moderate drinking—one drink per day, maximum—is crucial if you are trying to stay within your calorie budget. Alcohol is a dense source of calories. If you drink just three glasses of wine, you will be getting up to 375 calories without any nutrition whatsoever. Further, alcohol can actually block the absorption of important nutrients such as folate and other B vitamins.[2] So I stress this point: Drink only if it fits into your personal calorie budget *after* you have eaten your three meals and snacks—you need the nutrients these provide; the alcohol is superfluous.

Health and Alcohol

Benefits

Dozens of studies have demonstrated that drinking small amounts of alcohol every day reduces the risk of heart disease caused by blocked arteries by 10 to 15 percent.[3] This is because the ethanol in alcohol has two beneficial qualities. First, it increases good HDL cholesterol, which cuts down our bad LDL cholesterol plaques, allowing blood to flow to and from the heart more easily and preventing heart attacks. Second, it prevents blood platelets from clumping together and forming clots, which can cause strokes. These cardiovascular benefits come from all types of alcohol—beer, spirits, and wine.

TYPE	SERV. SIZE	ALCOHOL CONTENT	CALORIES PER SERV.	COMMENTS
Lite beer	12 oz	~3%	~90–100	A common serving of beer is a 16-oz pint; this is 1½ servings, even though it is served as 1.
Regular beer	12 oz	~5%	~150–200	
Lager	12 oz	4.9%	~180	
Wheat	12 oz	4.9%	~165	
Ale	12 oz	5.3%	~160	
Red wine	5 oz	Alcohol content of wine varies from 8–24% due to region (European are less alcoholic than domestic) and other factors (table wine has less than fortified wines)	~100–130	Size of glass and generosity of pours varies; a huge pour may have you drinking 1½ or 2 servings in one glass.
Cabernet	5 oz		~130	
Pinot Noir	5 oz		~120	
Merlot	5 oz		~120	
White wine	5 oz		~100–120	
Sauvignon Blanc	5 oz		~120	
Chardonnay	5 oz		~120	
Dry Riesling	5 oz		~110	
Rosé	5 oz		~100	
Champagne	5 oz		~100	
Dessert wine	3.5 oz		~165	
80-proof spirits (vodka, gin, rum, tequila, whiskey)	1.5 oz	40%	~100	Many bartenders eyeball rather than measure shots, so you may get a stronger drink with double the calories.
Proper cocktails*				In mixed drinks, the mixer you choose can contain lots of hidden calories.
Gin or vodka martini	varies		~150	
Gin & tonic	varies		~200	
Rum & Coke	varies		~200	
Vodka & orange juice	varies		~160	
Cosmopolitan	4 oz		~200	
Margarita or mojito	varies		~500	

*Serving sizes, alcohol content, and calories can vary widely based on pour and glass size.

So, what about the red wine hype? The jury is still out on the actual health benefits of red wine, but it is possible that red wine provides cancer-fighting antioxidants. The "good" components of red wine are found in the grape skins, which are left out of white wine. Animal studies have shown red wine and purple grape juice alike to have cardio-protective effects. However, there may also be something about the fermentation process that increases the flavonoid content of red wine over grape juice. The evidence is not conclusive, but enjoying a 5-ounce glass of your favorite California Pinot Noir at the end of the day may be minimally beneficial to your health, and it can certainly be a nice way to unwind.

While the occasional drink can provide a nice mental boost for most of us—a positive effect which should not be discounted—it is important to remember that alcohol is technically a depressant. Overindulging can lead to mood swings and possible anxiety and depression the next day. Have you ever woken up after a great night out and felt inexplicably down (not to mention ill)? It's because you essentially overdosed on a depressant substance. Alcohol must be used in moderation to reap the positive benefits without paying the price.

Risks

Although alcohol provides some health benefits, according to the CDC, it is the third leading cause of preventable death in the United States after smoking and obesity, mostly due to alcohol-related cancers and drunk driving. Regular alcohol use can cause liver disease or cancer, as well as cancer of the mouth, throat, esophagus, pancreas, breast, and colon. While this risk is different for every person, it is likely dose-dependent, meaning the more you drink, the higher your risk. One explanation is that alcohol could impair the liver's ability to filter out cancer-causing toxins. Another explanation is that alcohol increases the level of estrogen in the body, thereby putting women at greater risk for breast cancer.

Genetics also play a role in alcohol's risk profile. This is crucial information for you ladies with a family history of cancer, specifically breast cancer. Research suggests that even two alcoholic drinks (of any kind) per day could increase the risk of this disease by 50 percent in women with familial breast cancer.[4] This is why I say Healthy Habit #6 is optional. Now is the time to talk to your relatives and assess your family's history of disease to calculate your own risk/benefit profile for alcohol consumption.

Alcohol dependence is another danger of regular alcohol use. If you find yourself drinking more than seven drinks a week or otherwise occasionally indulging in binge drinking (defined as five or more drinks for males and four or more drinks for females over the course of about 2 hours) your chances of developing alcohol dependence increase. The Harvard School of Public Health's College Alcohol Study evidenced that binge drinking on American college campuses has become a serious issue.[5] As a nutritionist, I have seen an increased tendency to carry these binge drinking behaviors from college into adulthood, whereby a typical night on the town continues to include several drinks and a weekend is often formed around where and how to become intoxicated with friends, or even on a date. You should be aware that even occasional binge drinkers have higher mortality rates than those who drink moderately on a regular basis. When you consume three or more drinks in one sitting, you are at an increased risk for elevated serum triglycerides, or fat, in your bloodstream, because alcohol is metabolized like a fat in your body. This can cause coronary heart disease and so negates any of alcohol's positive cardio-protective effects.

Out on the Town

Knowing the benefits and risks of alcohol is important in making healthy choices. If you are heading out for the evening—either starting at happy hour or later on in the night—and it seems inevitable that you will indulge in more than one drink, here are some important strategies for keeping yourself from overdoing it:

- **Alternate every alcoholic drink with water.** Alcohol is a diuretic (makes you pee). It promotes urine production by reducing your anti-diuretic hormone and inhibiting your kidneys from conserving body water. Once you "break the seal" and start going to the bathroom, you should also start to drink water to compensate for the fluid you are losing.

- **Dilute your white wine by ordering a spritzer.** This is white wine mixed with a splash of seltzer water, which increases the portion of your drink while decreasing the alcohol and calorie content.

- **Order dry white wine** (*e.g.*, Sauvignon Blanc) **over a sweeter white** (*e.g.*, Riesling). Dry wines take longer to sip and typically contain fewer calories.

- **Opt for a higher-end version of your favorite spirit** (like vodka or tequila) **and drink it on the rocks.** With a twist of lemon or lime, it's a great alternative to a mixed drink. You'll save calories, and it will take longer to sip.

- **Go for diet tonic, diet soda, or seltzer water as a mixer.** This combats calorie (and sugar) intake in mixed drinks. But be sure to sip slowly: Recent research suggests that diet soda used as a mixer could increase the effects of alcohol intoxication; artificial sweeteners may cause alcohol to hit the bloodstream more quickly.[6]

- **Order a club soda with a splash of vodka.** It is extra light in calories and alcohol content, but will still give you the feeling that you are drinking something with some oomph.

- **Try a virgin mixed drink or sparkling seltzer water with lime.** If you've had enough partying but your friends haven't, no one has to know there is no alcohol in your glass. Besides, you'll have something to sip that will also help sober you up.

- **Stay away from novelty drinks.** Anything that is frozen; an unnatural shade of blue, green, or purple; comes with a sugared or salted rim; or includes little umbrellas or floating candies can contain as many calories as a meal! Save these for a tropical beach vacation.

Savvy Girl Tip

Instead of just boozing with your girls, sit at the bar and order appetizers with one glass of wine to split. The bartender will usually give you two glasses, each with about three-fourths of a regular glass so you will get almost a whole drink each (two glasses for the price of one) but also keep your alcohol and calories in check. Just make sure to leave your bartender a nice tip!

The Hangover

Maybe it was the never-ending wine glass at your book club, or simply a couple of cocktails without enough dinner. No matter how hard you try to be responsible, now and then all of us wind up suffering from a nasty hangover. Even more annoying, your symptoms seem to be more severe and persistent than when you were 21. Typical hangovers should abate within 8 to 24 hours after waking up, but you may feel dazed and confused for a couple days depending on how much damage you inflicted on yourself. Further, your hangover may hang on longer if you suffer from alcohol-induced insomnia. Have you ever woken up in the middle of the night after an evening out and been unable to go back to sleep? It's a symptom of alcohol withdrawal, and it can keep you from getting enough zzz's to "sleep it off." On the other hand, you may be someone who, once intoxicated, hits the pillow and snores through the night. Alcohol can cause your throat to relax, which may increase your tendency to snore and can even cause periodic cessation of breathing, or sleep apnea. This often leads to fatigue the next day because you haven't gotten enough oxygen throughout the night.

Here are some tips to help you curb a hangover, especially when you have to be a functioning adult at work in the morning:

◆ **Chug as much water as you possibly can before bed.** Do it again in the morning when you wake up. Alcohol dries you out, and rehydrating is key to staving off electrolyte imbalances, dizziness, headaches, and lightheadedness.

◆ **Eat before you go to bed.** (This is the only time I will actually advise this.) Something bland with complex carbohydrates like toast, cereal, crackers, or pretzels will help soak up stomach acid, relieve nausea, and stabilize your blood sugar. Because eating is crucial to eliminating a hangover, and excess drinking means you have already consumed too many calories, overindulging should be infrequent (no more than once a month at most).

◆ **Do your best to make sure anything more than one drink a night does not become a habit.** While eating before bed is better than getting sick from binge drinking, even one or two drinks can increase your appetite and reduce your ability to withstand temptation (in more ways than one).

◆ **Wash your face and brush your teeth before you go to bed.** Even if you really don't want to. This will alleviate some of the disgusting taste brought on by "cotton mouth" and you will surely feel fresher when you wake up (if you don't look like you have been punched in the eye from your running mascara).

◆ **Try a sports drink like Gatorade** (especially the new low-calorie G2) **in the morning to replenish your electrolytes.**

◆ **Take a daily multivitamin/mineral supplement *with* your breakfast** (not on an empty stomach). This ensures that you aren't lacking important nutrients—not only can alcohol leach nutrients from your body, but some girls forgo food for alcohol to save calories.

◆ **Try to eat some fruit.** An apple or a banana is a good option. The potassium in the banana will help stabilize your electrolyte levels, and the fibrous apple will help you detox (*i.e.*, go to the bathroom).

◆ **For a pounding headache, opt for Advil.** Stay away from Tylenol (acetaminophen), as it can cause serious liver damage when mixed with alcohol. Also steer clear of aspirin, which can be a gastric irritant when paired with booze.

◆ **For an upset stomach, chew on a Tums to neutralize acid.** As an added bonus, this antacid will also give you a shot of calcium.

◆ **Go to the gym in the morning before work.** Exercise can mitigate the effects of drinking.

Reduce and Quit Smoking

Before I finish this chapter, I wanted to deal with the cocktail's common and often more addictive companion: the cigarette. By now we all know that smoking increases the risk of heart disease, stroke, cancer, respiratory problems, and yes, death. Long-term smokers are also more likely to develop premature wrinkling, lose teeth, and get this—their hair is up to four times more likely to turn prematurely gray![7,8] And this is to say nothing of the stench that permeates every smoker's wardrobe, furniture, and hair. Thank goodness so many cities have finally banned smoking in bars and restaurants—this has gone a long way toward helping "social smokers" kick the habit. Here are some smoking cessation tools if you are interested. Remember, defeating this addiction may be the best thing you can do to prevent disease (and death). As your nutritionist, I would rather see you gain five pounds after quitting than continue smoking.

◆ In 2007, Duke University administered a questionnaire to 209 smokers. It was found that caffeinated and alcoholic beverages enhance the taste of cigarettes. On the other hand, dairy products, fruits and vegetables, juice, and water actually worsen the taste.[9] So, the next time you want a cigarette, try pairing it with a glass of milk or OJ instead of a glass of wine and see how palatable those cigarettes really are.

◆ Dr. Adrianne Cantor, an internal medicine doctor in Philadelphia (and my sister), often sees young women about their efforts to quit smoking. She says that different approaches work for different people, so some will have to try a couple of strategies to quit for good. In terms of medical intervention, she recommends options such as (1) nicotine replacement therapy, like the patch or nicotine gum; (2) prescription medication available from your physician; (3) stress-reducing exercise such as aerobic activity or yoga; and (4) alternative modalities such as hypnosis. Ask your doctor about these different options.

- Try hypnosis—visit www.AmericanHypnosisClinic.com. In a Massachusetts study of 67 patients with heart disease, half of those given hypnotherapy to quit smoking remained smoke-free after six months, whereas only a quarter of those in the "cold-turkey" arm of the study maintained smoking cessation.[10] It can be a good option.

- Visit www.SmokeFree.gov to find more ideas about how to beat your nicotine addiction. And get as much support from family and friends as possible—this is a very tough feat, but you can do it.

Now that we've gone over two of our most common "fixes," I hope you feel equipped to make healthy decisions about your recreational choices. My advice is to take Healthy Habit #6 with a grain of salt and use this as an excuse to look into your family's medical history if you haven't done so already. Social drinking can be a normal part of our lives, but just like staying out in the sun too long, it's a habit we may regret in twenty years if we overindulge.

Next, we deal with dinner—just the thought of it gives me a natural high.

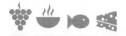 ## CHEW ON THIS!

To quit smoking, hypnotists conjure up the thing you hate most about your dirty habit. For example, you've always hated the residual smell of stale ash all over your clothing and hands. When you wake up and go for that butt, all you will be able to imagine is that stench and smoking becomes a no-go. Pretty cool, right?

PROFILE

Scribing and Imbibing

Ah, the life of a writer. Lola, one of my favorite clients, would wake up every morning and stumble directly to her computer. It would boot up as she brewed a pot of coffee and her writing began with her first sip. She'd proceed to work through the day in her sunny little apartment (yes, in her pajamas). Sounds pretty sweet, right? The only problem was that after working at home, alone, all day long, Lola was always rarin' to go out and get social at night. And, since she lived in the city, scheduling a week full of social events was never an issue. Lola loved her wine, and some nights her dirty martinis. Because she had the luxury of sleeping in and making her own hours, a mellow dinner with the girls often turned into a night of heavy drinking and overindulging.

THE SOLUTION

Lola needed to learn how to practice restraint. The first thing we did was make her aware of just how much she was drinking in a week. I had her track the frequency of her alcohol use—and just seeing her habits on paper was a shock to her system. We set a limit for her of five to seven drinks per week. I had her get in the habit of choosing in advance two alcohol-free nights, three nights of enjoying one drink, and one or two nights where she could indulge in a couple of drinks more freely. By keeping track of how frequently she was drinking, Lola has been able to naturally keep herself in check—and save a lot of calories (and hangovers) in the process. What's more, she has noticed that she no longer wakes up feeling depressed or anxious in the mornings.

Chapter 11

Restaurant "Weak"

IN MY PRACTICE, I've noticed that women who work full-time tend to eat about 40 percent of their total daily calories after 5 p.m. By now I hope you are on my bandwagon of eating throughout the day so you won't arrive at dinner feeling famished (or hung over from happy hour) and can **eat in the range of 500 to 600 calories for dinner.** I'll take you through several dining-out scenarios and show you how to make smart choices, whether you usually eat out with clients, go on a hot midweek date, or have a standing Thursday night dinner with girlfriends. Though restaurant dining offers a multitude of options, I recommend Healthy Habit #7: Use eating out as an opportunity to eat fish. As you know, fish is an extremely important part of your diet as it is a main source of heart-healthy omega-3 fatty acids. I want you to try to eat two or more servings of fish every week.

You're probably aware that restaurant meals are laden with hidden calories—they often contain more butter, oil, cream, and cheese than you might expect (or could imagine). And then, of course, there are the huge portion sizes. So how can you practice your healthy habits while dining out during the workweek? Here are a few tips to help you navigate this potential minefield:

- ◆ **Save the true indulgences for special occasions.** It's fine to splurge on a special meal every now and then. Just remember, it's your daily habits that matter.

- ◆ **Plan ahead.** Before you leave the office, check out www.MenuPages.com or the restaurant's Web site and take a look at an online menu to decide what you are going to order before getting to the table.

- ◆ **Eat your afternoon snack.** Ordering appetizers or eating bread as soon as you are seated will be less tempting if you are not ravenous.

- ◆ **Skip the breadbasket.** Intercept the waiter before he puts it down and ask that he skip your table. Save those calories for a delicious baguette dipped in olive oil over the weekend and really savor it.

- ◆ **Make difficult choices.** Before you start eating, decide whether you are going to have dessert *or* a cocktail (or neither). Making this decision up front will help you avoid temptation when the various menus are passed around.

- ◆ **Always drink water.** This should be your main source of hydration with dinner.

- ◆ **Use the Plate Method.** As a general rule, half of your plate should contain nonstarchy veggies, a quarter of your plate, 3 to 5 ounces of lean protein, and the last quarter, about ½ cup

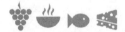 CHEW ON THIS!

A group of researchers from the University of Memphis studied the effect of eating out on diet quality in 129 premenopausal women. They found that those who reported eating out a greater number of times per week had higher calorie, fat, and sodium intakes but did not get as much fiber or calcium, even in the extra energy consumed.[1]

of a starchy food—like rice or sweet potato. Use these guide-lines when ordering your entrée and choosing sides.

- **Try soup.** When in doubt, start with a vegetable, chicken, or beef broth–based soup (as opposed to a cream or coconut milk–based) to fill you up without lots of calories.

- **Order half or appetizer-sized portions.** Ask your waiter to divide your meal in half and pack it up *before* it is served. (My 93-year-old Mommom has been doing this for years . . . I used to think it was embarrassing, but now I have to say it is sort of chic.)

- **Order two appetizers instead of an app and a main course.** Start with a salad that contains a little bit of fat (it will be very satiating). Then go for seafood, shrimp cocktail, ceviche, or a (broiled) crab cake. Trust me, on a random Tuesday night, you will feel better and sleep better if you eat less before you go to bed.

- **Be politely picky.** Request substitutions in cooking method or ingredient when you can. It's the twenty-first century—people ask for fried fish to be grilled, sautéed vegetables to be steamed, or brown rice in lieu of white all the time. Remember: The goal is to look hip (not hippy) in your designer jeans.

- **Be inquisitive.** Ask your waiter questions if you are unsure of what is in the meal, how it is cooked, or how big the portion is. A key question to ask: "Is it made with cream?" If the answer is yes, modify or make another selection.

- **Have sauce on the side.** Ask your waiter for salad dressing and heavy sauces on the side so you can eat what you want and not more. Dip your fork into the sauce first and then spear your food.

- **Steer clear here.** Avoid menu items that include words like *fried, fritto, fritti, crunchy, sautéed,* and anything in which a main ingredient is listed as *cheese, coconut milk,* or *butter.*

- **Choose these.** Aim to order options that contain words like steamed, raw, grilled, tomato-based, poached (unless it is butter poached), broiled, or roasted.

- **Take a breather.** In the middle of your meal, put down the fork for a few minutes to give your stomach time to feel full, and make sure to drink some water. It's also a great time to stop focusing on eating and give your dining companions your full attention.

- **A little left is right.** Leave a little something on your plate—like one last good bite. It will pay off in the long run. Don't worry about wasting food—as I stated before, there are 3,900 calories per person available in this country every day, so plate waste is necessary to prevent our whole country from becoming obese.

Now let's go over some common dining-out scenarios that you are likely to face during the week.

Scenario #1: A Client Dinner—The Steak House

Remember, when it comes to business dinners, don't succumb to the temptation to order *more* food just because you're not picking up the check. Instead, view it as an opportunity to indulge in higher-quality, healthy food and enjoy it to the fullest.

- A steak house provides a perfect opportunity to incorporate Healthy Habit #7. Choose from the nice selection of fresh grilled or broiled fish such as bass, trout, tuna, and salmon.

- Go for the steamed or grilled lobster—a great treat, especially when you're not paying. A 6-ounce serving has about 160 calories and is a great source of omega-3s and protein. Just be sure to stay away from the warm butter on the side—try lemon and cocktail sauce instead.

- Eat appetizers such as a shrimp or crab cocktail or tuna tartare as your main course. These are usually entrée-sized and provide lean protein and omega-3s. Order a small side salad as an appetizer if you want two courses.

◆ Modify your salad order if necessary. Ask them to hold the cheese or croutons, put the dressing on the side, or substitute vinaigrette for a creamy dressing.

◆ If you decide to indulge in a steak, go for the leanest cuts of meat. Always ask your waiter what the leanest cut available is. Try a steak with the word *loin*—like top sirloin or tenderloin (which includes filet mignon), or *round*—like eye of round or top round. The highly bioavailable iron and zinc make steak a healthy treat once in a while.

◆ A healthy serving of meat is 4 to 6 ounces; beware of 12-plus-ounce steaks. Order the "mini" or "petite" filet and/or eat half and take the rest home to slice on a salad for lunch the next day or else for your dog (or your other half), or share with a colleague at the table. While this doesn't sound like very much, beef is rich and filling and a 4-ounce portion is packed with ample amounts of iron, zinc, B vitamins, phosphorus, and niacin.

◆ Stay away from Kobe beef, any kind of ribs, and bacon during the week—all of these choices contain an excessive amount of saturated fat.

◆ Beware of steakhouse specialty or "house" sauces. These are typically cheese or butter-based and, at a good steak house, largely superfluous given the high quality of meat you are consuming. Stick to salt, pepper, and steak rubs.

◆ Choose nutritious sides. Most steakhouses offer roasted or steamed veggies like asparagus, broccoli, and Brussels sprouts. If you order the steamed (not "creamed") spinach or a baked potato, be sure to ask for the butter/oil on the side—or better yet, not at all. Use lemon or the juice from the steak to flavor your food instead.

Scenario #2: Take-Out at the Office—Sushi

It's 8 p.m. and you're still at work frantically trying to meet a deadline. I know you feel like a desperate desk-wife, but again, do not order more just because it's on your company or you want to comfort yourself. The research is clear—when you are served more, you will eat more.[2] It is important to order just enough food to satisfy your hunger and no more—otherwise you will likely polish off way more calories than you need.

- ◆ Start with a healthy appetizer. Miso soup is filling and only about 50 calories; edamame is a good source of soy protein at about 125 calories; seaweed salad has roughly 70 calories and contains many minerals from the sea and vitamin K; and steamed shrimp shumai are about 100 to 150 calories per order and contain protein and omega-3s.

- ◆ A green salad with ginger dressing is always a good option. Just ask for the dressing on the side so that your salad isn't soggy by the time it arrives.

- ◆ Incorporate Healthy Habit #7 again—go for the fresh fish! Sashimi is lower-cal (about 30 calories per piece) than sushi (about 65 calories) because it comes without rice.

- ◆ Stay away from fried Japanese foods like tempura, which is battered and fried, "crunchies" in your sushi roll (these are

 CHEW ON THIS!

Chew on this: In a 2004 study, customers at a cafeteria were tricked: Half were given a typical, full-sized portion of a baked pasta dish, while the other half got 50 percent more of the same entree. Unknowingly, the customers who got the bigger plates ate about 43 percent more calories. They also ate more bread to soak it all up![3]

---

tempura pieces), and the spider roll, which is typically made with deep-fried crab.

◆ Steer clear of too much teriyaki—a glaze that is typically made with a lot of salt and sugar. If you want the grilled teriyaki chicken, ask for the sauce on the side and use as a dip.

◆ It's easy to get carried away with rolls, which can be deceptively high in calories. Try to order no more than one sushi roll per meal and ask for brown rice when available. Alternatively, you can ask the sushi chefs to go "light on the rice." Here are rough calorie counts for popular rolls—make sure your order falls within your calorie budget:

- Spicy salmon or tuna roll: 450 to 500 calories

- California roll: 350 calories

- Shrimp avocado roll: 350 calories

- Vegetable roll: 250 calories

◆ Try hibachi chicken, salmon, shrimp, scallops, or beef. It is basically lean protein in soy-based sauce. Whenever possible, always ask for low-sodium soy sauces to accompany your meal.

◆ Foods described as "spicy" are often made with spicy mayonnaise. If you've gotta have it, ask for this high-cal condiment on the side and add a touch to your roll with a chopstick. Wasabi is a better choice as it adds the same kick with virtually no calories. Pickled ginger (the pink stuff) is another good option—low-cal and good for your digestion.

Scenario #3: Girls' Night Out—The French Bistro

If you are anything like me, dressing up to go out to dinner with your girlfriends or simply meeting after work to de-stress and chat it up is a highlight of the week. But did you know that your girl group could be affecting your weight? A 2007 research study published by the *New England Journal of Medicine* tracked more than 12,000 people and established that obesity spreads within social networks.[4] One explanation for this phenomenon is that when a friend, spouse, or sibling gains weight, you more readily accept weight gain in yourself; or, stated another way, when they pig out, you are more likely to gorge yourself too (who wants to eat a brownie sundae alone?). So take note of your social scene. If your girls are craving *moules frites* but you know it will blow your calorie budget, don't feel pressured to ruin your diet for their sake. You can always meet them for a drink afterward, or better yet, use one of these strategies to join in the fun without paying a hefty price.

◆ Decide ahead of time to indulge in *either* the breadbasket, a glass of wine, *or* dessert—and enjoy it to the fullest. Remember, too much variety leads to overeating.

◆ Skip the high-calorie French onion soup and instead go for the raw bar—a shrimp cocktail or raw oysters are always delicious and can count toward Healthy Habit #7—eat fish!

◆ For your entrée, try fish native to the bistro: skate, red snapper, or cod. Ask your waiter to fillet it to remove the bones and eat it with plenty of fresh lemon juice.

◆ Try a *salade niçoise*. This is a classic at most bistros and the tuna is a good source of lean protein and heart-healthy omega-3s. Make sure to order your vinaigrette dressing on the side.

◆ Go for the mussels as your main entrée. Skip the *moules marinières*, made with white wine and cream, and instead go for the *moules provençales*, made with white wine and tomato base. Also, skip the fries (*frites*) that often accompany this dish and enjoy two pieces of bread to soak up the sauce instead.

◆ If you are not feeling like fish, I love the chicken paillard salad, which typically is thin grilled chicken breast topped with yummy salad greens. Again, order salad dressing on the side.

◆ Skip the high-calorie quiche, a bistro staple typically made with plenty of cream and butter. If you are feeling like eggs, go for the omelet and ask for egg whites and veggies.

◆ A side of veggies is always a great choice, but be aware that seemingly healthy sides like sautéed spinach can be full of oil or butter. Ask your waiter for steamed instead and eat them with lemon juice. Or substitute a mixed green salad for any side, and *always* in lieu of the fries.

◆ If you girls want dessert, order one dessert for the table and take two rounded spoonfuls.

Scenario #4: Date Night—Italian

These days, dinner dates are no longer for Saturday night only. If you're dating, you are probably eating out more often than not. This can be a big drain on your calorie budget. But it should also be an opportunity for you to have a little fun. (BTW: If you aren't dating—get online now!) Here are some suggestions for how to order a healthy date night dinner:

◆ Italy is renowned for its seafood dishes, so go for Healthy Habit #7 and order fresh fish and shellfish for your main course. Just be careful with your sauces—you can always substitute if needed.

- When it comes to sauces, go for red. Tomato-based sauces are always a better choice than cream or meat sauces such as alfredo, vodka, carbonara, or bolognese.

- Ask for half or side portions of pasta—or better yet, split a pasta entrée with your date.

- Avoid pasta dishes that feature cheese as a main ingredient, such as manicotti, lasagna, or ravioli.

- Fill up on the minestrone soup as an appetizer—it's hearty and full of fiber and protein. In fact, you can eat it as a main course with a salad starter.

- Italian food is great for sharing. If you're dying to try the caprese salad or the grilled calamari, order one appetizer and share with your date.

- When it comes to pizza, go for thin crust loaded with veggies (fresh, roasted, and baked), sprinkle with red pepper flakes and freshly ground pepper, and eat a slice or two with a side salad. Avoid deep-dish crusts, lots of cheese, and oily toppings like pepperoni and sausage.

Other Ethnic Fare

Part of the fun of dining out is enjoying foods from different cultures. As usual, and particularly when you are less familiar with the items on the menu, it is crucial to solicit the help of your waiter to better understand how dishes are prepared, the main ingredients, and the portion sizes—each restaurant is a little different. Remember, they can usually modify when asked. Turn to pages 132–133 for a chart of common ethnic food that will help you navigate the menu the next time you dine out or order in.

Dessert

Uh-oh, here comes the dessert menu. To open or not to open—that is the question. My advice is to save decadent sweets for special occasions (your birthday, the holidays, etc.). However, so you do not feel deprived Monday through Friday, I'd like to advocate a *once-a-week shared dessert*. If and when you are at a delicious restaurant with friends or a sweetheart, go ahead and indulge in one Decadent Do per week. This should consist of no more than two rounded spoonfuls of whatever your party decides to order. Enjoy it without guilt. Otherwise, order a decaf espresso or cappuccino with skim milk and call it a night.

As much fun as it is to spend the evening dining out, we working girls can also appreciate a night in, chilling on the sofa. Whether you love to cook or can barely heat up a can of soup, next we'll delve into why dining in can be one of the healthiest habits around.

CUISINE	TRY
CHINESE	Hot tea
	Soup: wonton or hot & sour
	Steamed dumplings
	Steamed brown rice
	Steamed shrimp, chicken, or vegetable dishes
	Sauce on the side (they're all full of oil, so moderate)
	Ordering one dish fewer than there are people at the table
	Eating with chopsticks
THAI	Thai salad
	Broth-based soup
	Chicken satay (easy on the peanut sauce)
	Thai lettuce wraps
	Fresh spring (summer) rolls
	Dishes with steamed or grilled veggies, shrimp, or fish
	Sharing curry entrees
	Sauce on the side
INDIAN	Raita (shredded cucumbers, tomatoes, yogurt)
	Sambal (spicy chopped tomato and onion)
	Roti (whole wheat bread baked in clay oven)
	Chutneys (made from herbs, spices, coconut)
	Tandoori chicken or fish (baked in a clay oven with spice rub, no sauce)
	Dal (legume- and lentil-based dish)
	Sambhar (lentil curry)
	Vegetarian options
	Sharing curry entrees
	$\frac{1}{2}$ cup of rice or bread (not both)
MEXICAN	Black and pinto beans
	Pulled chicken
	Fresh salsa, picante, guacamole
	Fresh veggies
	Soft whole wheat or corn tortillas or tacos
	Salad on a plate, not in a fried bowl
	Make-your-own fajitas (limit yourself to one tortilla)

Fried appetizers like egg rolls, dumplings, or the pupu platter

Fried rice or fried noodles

Items described as crispy, golden brown, or sweet and sour—these are all fried

Kung Pao and General Tso's Chicken

Dishes with MSG (ask your waiter)

Peking Duck with skin

Fried spring rolls

Oil-laden carbohydrate bomb Pad Thai

Dishes soaked in coconut milk

Excess white rice

Samosas (fried dumplings)

Butter naan (white flour flatbread with a ton of butter)

Paratha (heavy bread)

Thick curries made with spices, butter, and yogurt like Tikka Masala and Butter Chicken

Makhani (butter)

Ghee (clarified butter)

Malai, rasmalai (thick cream)

Fried chips, nachos, fried tortilla shells

Excess cheese

Sour cream

Refried beans

Dishes with these words: charro beans (refried), con queso (with cheese), chimichanga (fried burrito), or chalupa (deep-fried tortilla)

Quesadillas

PROFILE

Salt Lick

Wendy worked for a few years as an editor fresh out of college, then went back to business school. Upon graduation, she decided to put her writing and business skills together to work as a literary agent. Wendy made the right choice. She eventually garnered a great track record of matching writers with publishers.

Her biggest grievance was that her long workdays were typically topped off by working dinners out. Wendy felt like she knew how to navigate a menu and order the right things—soups and salads, two appetizers in lieu of a main, and she routinely chose one glass of wine instead of bread or dessert. Nevertheless, she felt bloated many mornings when she woke up after a working dinner. Her eyes felt swollen and her rings were tight. And on these days, she also felt headachey but didn't think one glass of wine was enough to make her feel hung over.

THE SOLUTION

When Wendy came to my office, we did a 24-hour recall in which she recounted everything she had eaten the day before. The first half of Wendy's day seemed quite healthy, but I quickly saw a bad trend developing as her day progressed. Wendy's afternoon snack consisted of 1 ounce of salted mixed nuts. Dinner was spent at a steakhouse, where she started the night with a cocktail at the bar accompanied by a few olives. Then she skipped the breadbasket and ordered a broth-based soup for her appetizer. She ordered the grilled halibut with sauce on the side and used salt to bring out the flavor. She had steamed spinach, again with salt, as a side. Calorie for calorie, Wendy was on target, but in terms of sodium intake—she was definitely overdoing it.

To say nothing of its negative effect on blood pressure, salt can be bloating for certain individuals who are "salt sensitive." Wendy fit this bill—so even though she was doing a great job of eating out healthfully in terms of calories and fat, she was overloading on salt. I wanted Wendy to aim for a goal of less than 2,300 mg of sodium per day, which is equal to a little less than 1 teaspoon of salt. The first strategy I stressed was absolute: No more salting restaurant food, especially before trying it. Other strategies we discussed included eating only unsalted nuts, using lemon juice and pepper to flavor veggies and fish, asking for food to be prepared without salt or MSG, drinking water throughout dinner to dilute salt, and eating fruits (bananas, melon, peaches) high in potassium during the day to counteract sodium buildup.

Wendy reports feeling much less bloated. In her words, she no longer wakes up feeling as if she spent the night "on the salt lick."

CHAPTER 12

Home Body

DOES IT FEEL LIKE you never get an evening to yourself? For some working women, staying in can actually be a greater privilege than dining out at a fantastic restaurant—being surrounded by rich food and having to be "on" all the time can get old. Not only can eating in save you calories and money, it can be an excellent way to de-stress after a long day, especially if you like to cook. As such, I would like to introduce Healthy Habit #8: Make a resolution to cook dinner at least once a week (more often is even better). A recent study of the eating habits of young adults (18 to 23) revealed that those who purchased and prepared their own foods were more likely to meet dietary recommendations for fat, calcium, fruits, vegetables, and whole grain intake.[1] However, the respondents who didn't cook (and who had an inferior diet) cited lack of time or culinary skills as reasons they didn't make their own meals.

With this in mind, I have put together a list of quick-and-healthy weeknight dinners. This is not a recipe guide *per se*; rather, I want to provide you with some very simple ideas and guidelines so you can quickly make a delicious dinner using wholesome, nutritious foods. I promise that you don't need to be a four-star chef and you won't need to spend hours in the kitchen to prepare these simple meals. And if you are consistently stocking your cupboard, refrigerator, and freezer with my original list of staple foods, you should be all set to make these meals with very little extra shopping.

Easy Weeknight Meals

Main Courses

1. *Broiled Chicken Breast:* Rinse a 6-ounce chicken breast (per person) in the sink, place it on a cookie sheet or broiling pan, and sprinkle with salt and pepper. Set your oven to high broil (500°F), and place your pan on the top rack or in the broiler drawer. Cook for about 5 to 7 minutes per side. Note: If you want to marinate your raw chicken, let it marinate in one part low-sodium soy sauce (one tablespoon per breast), one part brown sugar (one tablespoon per breast), and a pinch of garlic powder for at least 15 minutes; then cook as above.

2. *Baked (a.k.a. Roasted) Chicken:* You might be afraid to cook an entire chicken, but it is super-easy and can provide you with meals for three days. Preheat oven to 375°F. Rinse the chicken inside and out (toss the bag of giblets if it's

 CHEW ON THIS!

Studies show that mothers who engage in behaviors such as drinking meal replacements (like Slim-Fast) while the rest of the family eats dinner together instigate disordered eating in their children.[2] To be a good role model for your family (presently or in the future), learn how to eat well and enjoy food together.

inside) and place it in a shallow pan. Bake for about 1½ to 2 hours, or until the internal temperature is 170°F and the juices run clear. Remove and let it rest about 10 minutes before carving. You can always pick up a rotisserie chicken at the grocery store instead, but it is pricier. Eat the chicken plain or pull it off the bone to toss it into a soup or pasta dish, put on a sandwich for a quick workday lunch, or mix with taco seasoning to make chicken tacos.

3. *Broiled Salmon:* Buy about 6 to 8 ounces of raw fish per person—it shrinks with cooking. Rinse it in the sink, lay it on a foil-lined broiling pan or a cookie sheet, and sprinkle with pepper, Old Bay Seasoning, and lemon. Set your oven to high broil (500°F) and place your pan on the top rack or in the broiler drawer. Cook for about 10 minutes and check. Depending on how big/thick your piece is, you may need 5 more minutes. If it is a really thick piece of fish, after 15 minutes, lower the rack so the top of your fish does not get too burned (though it is nice for the top to be crispy and partially blackened). You can cook Chilean sea bass the exact same way.

4. *Pan-Fried Tilapia:* Lightly coat a nonstick frying pan with cooking spray and heat to medium-high. Fry fish on each side for about 3 minutes. Sprinkle with lemon, salt, and pepper and top with salsa. This pairs nicely with black beans—pop open a can and eat them on the side.

5. *Scrambled Eggs with Veggies:* One egg has approximately 80 calories, but the white part accounts for only about 20 calories and is full of protein. The yolk contains up to 60 calories and has all the egg's fat and cholesterol, but also the most vitamins and minerals (including iron). Try using the ratio of 1 whole egg for every 2 egg whites. Whisk eggs

with a splash of nonfat milk, salt, and pepper. Lightly coat a frying pan with cooking spray and heat to medium. Add fresh or frozen veggies of your choice to the pan and sauté briefly. Pour in egg mixture and scramble until eggs are soft but not runny. Top with salsa or hot sauce and serve with whole wheat toast.

Savvy Girl Tip

It's tempting to sample as you cook—and those extra calories add up! When preparing a meal, try chewing gum to keep from nibbling.

6. *Whole Wheat Pasta with Veggie Marinara:* Cook pasta per package directions. Preheat a shallow pan on medium heat. Toss in fresh or frozen veggies—try spinach, broccoli, grated zucchini, diced peppers, onions, and/or fresh tomatoes—and cover with a jarred tomato sauce or a can of diced tomatoes. Simmer for 5 to 7 minutes. Serve over pasta, sprinkling with fresh grated parmesan cheese.

7. *Whole Wheat Pasta with Turkey Meat Sauce:* Cook pasta per package directions. Heat 1 tablespoon of extra virgin olive oil in a frying pan, and add turkey, making sure to stir it until it changes from pink to beige. Then drain the liquid. Cover with a jarred tomato sauce or a can of diced tomatoes and simmer for 5 to 10 minutes. Serve over pasta, sprinkling with fresh grated parmesan cheese.

8. *Quick Mexican Bowls:* Cook brown rice per package directions. Heat up a can of black or pinto beans and open a jar of salsa. If you have pulled chicken or cooked ground turkey meat, mix with taco seasoning. Slice an avocado; chop fresh lettuce; grate some sharp cheddar; and chop up some cilantro. Serve layered in individual bowls. Skipping the tortilla can save you upwards of 300 calories without sacrificing flavor.

9. *Stir-Fried Vegetables with or without Tofu or Shrimp:*
Make an easy marinade—mix low-sodium soy sauce and
brown sugar (add garlic and ginger if you have it). Wash
and chop veggies—use anything you have in your fridge
veggie drawer. Preheat frying pan to medium high, add a
splash of olive oil, and add the veggies and the marinade.
Cook until veggies are brightly colored but still crunchy
(about 7 to 10 minutes). Add slightly thawed frozen
cooked shrimp or cubed firm tofu for the last 5 minutes,
and serve.

10. *Homemade Tuna Salad:* Open an individual can of tuna
packed in water (about two ounces), drain, and dump the
contents into a bowl. Add 1 tablespoon of low-fat or fat-
free mayonnaise, 1 chopped celery stick, and 1 or 2
chopped pickles. Add salt and pepper to taste. Serve with a
piece of whole wheat toast or an English muffin, and top
with tomato if desired.

11. *Homemade BLT:* Toast two pieces of whole wheat bread,
spread ¼ of an avocado on one side, and top with 3 strips
of cooked turkey bacon, lettuce, and tomato.

12. *Easy Homemade Soups (see Chapter 8):* These can make
great dinners as well, accompanied by an easy salad or a
piece of whole wheat toast.

Now that we have our entrees down, let's focus on some
super-easy and healthy side dishes that you are sure to love.

Sides

1. *Roasted Root Vegetables:* Wash and prepare any combo of
sweet potatoes (wash and scrub, leave the skins on, and cut
into wedges), beets (peel with a potato peeler and cut into
fourths), turnips (peel with a potato peeler and cut into

fourths), peeled small onions or shallots, and carrots (use baby carrots or peel and cut a big carrot into pieces). Preheat oven to 400°F. Place veggies in a shallow pan and lightly coat with extra virgin olive oil, salt, and pepper. Bake for about an hour or a little longer if necessary. Veggies should be caramelized and soft when poked with a fork.

2. *Roasted Brussels Sprouts and Pine Nuts:* Wash Brussels sprouts, remove any outer, damaged leaves, and cut in half. Preheat oven to 375°F. Place sprouts in a shallow pan and lightly coat with extra virgin olive oil, lemon juice (if you have it), and salt and pepper. Stir and bake for about 40 minutes. Add pine nuts and cook for another 20 minutes. Sprouts and nuts should be caramelized and browned.

3. *Roasted Asparagus:* Wash asparagus and trim the stems. Preheat oven to 375°F. Place asparagus in a shallow pan and lightly coat with extra virgin olive oil, salt, and pepper. Bake for about 15 minutes.

4. *Steamed Vegetables:* Fill a pot with about 1½ inches of water (to just under the steamer). Place steamer basket in pot and turn heat to high. Add chopped veggies, cover, and cook until veggies turn brighter in color but are still crunchy, about 6 minutes (try green beans, asparagus, broccoli, or cabbage).

5. *Baked Potato:* Pierce medium potato with a fork a couple times. Preheat oven to 400°F. Bake for 60 minutes for a white potato or 45 for a sweet potato or yam.

6. *Starches:* Don't stop at brown rice and whole wheat pasta— try bulgur, quinoa, lentils, and couscous. Get creative with your grains and follow the easy directions on the package.

Frozen Dinners

Generally I am not a big fan of frozen meals because they tend to be highly processed and full of fat and sodium. However, I think the following selections are worth trying if you have not already. They are preportioned, widely available at most grocery stores, and handy to have available in your freezer. These dinners define cheap eats and run you in the 250- to 350-calorie range. If you can, add your own side salad or green veggie to bulk up your meal and add even more nutrients.

1. *Kashi Frozen Entrees*—All varieties emphasize whole grains, vegetables, and lean protein, and they actually taste fresh once you cook them. Kashi offers interesting tastes such as Black Bean Mango.

2. *Amy's Organic*—Organic, vegetarian, and kids love them too. Her lasagna is great, and the burritos made with whole grain tortillas are also popular.

3. *Lean Cuisine*—Go for the Spa Cuisine (in the light blue boxes). These emphasize whole grains like whole-wheat pasta and brown rice and are made with organic ingredients. I like the Chicken Pecan.

4. *Weight Watchers Smart Ones*—These will help you stay within your calorie budget. Try the Fruit Inspirations line, like the Orange Sesame Chicken.

5. *Healthy Choice*—Sample the Café Steamers line—the veggies are actually very crisp. The Chicken Marsala is delicious.

Late-Night Eating

Dinner's done—time to say good night to the kitchen, right? For most of us, it's not that easy. Too often, sitting on the sofa and watching TV leads to an uncontrollable urge to eat some more.

Let's address the affliction that is late-night eating.

Without fail, every client, and many a friend, asks me about late-night eating. A lot of women are very clean eaters during the day and socially, but cannot control their urges when left alone at night with a kitchen full of food. Contrary to popular opinion, the calories you eat right before bed are *not* more likely to turn to fat on your body than the calories you eat throughout the day.[3] However, eating after 9 p.m. can be dangerous, because at this point, you have probably already eaten your three meals and two snacks and therefore have most likely used up your calorie budget for the day. Moreover, you are probably inclined to choose a sugary, high-fat snack late at night, not a celery stick.

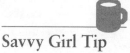

This is a time when it is important to understand the difference between hunger and appetite. Some late-night snackers are actually hungry. They rush through the day without enough sustenance and actually need calories at night. In this scenario, it is okay to complete your calorie budget through late-night eating. However, it is no fun to go to bed feeling stuffed, and lying down with a full stomach can cause heartburn, which makes it more difficult to fall asleep. I would rather see you eat your calories via healthy meals and snacks consistently throughout the day—and this would end your nighttime food cravings.

On the other hand, a lot of my clients are not hungry at all when they start to munch at 10 p.m. They have eaten all the calories in their budget, and late-night eating is a matter of pure appetite, not hunger. I like to offer these women the following strategies or diversions to curb a false appetite:

◆ Brush your teeth, chew gum, suck on a mint, put on a whitening strip, or apply a face mask

- Luxuriate in a bubble bath
- Stretch, do yoga poses, do sit-ups—go to Amazon.com and order a workout, yoga, or stretching DVD
- Go for a walk around the block—this is an especially good strategy if you have a dog or a friend/partner to accompany you
- Call someone
- Clean your apartment
- Partake in your favorite hobby—search iTunes for new music and make mixed CDs for your friends, knit, read, scrapbook, organize your digital pictures online, stalk people on Facebook, etc.
- Do something other than just watching TV, especially if you know that TV time is a catalyst for your overeating.

If you have a problem with late-night eating, do not, under any circumstances, have boxes of cookies or candy, donuts, full-fat ice cream, or other high-calorie junk in your house—these temptations are just too hard to resist. Try to stock up on some low-calorie snacks to munch when you're feeling the urge—think fruit, lo-cal hot drinks, Jell-O, and skim milk.

Strategies aside, late-night eating happens to all of us. Maybe you threw a dinner party at your house and end up polishing off

 **CHEW ON THIS!**

The brain has two neurophysiological systems—homeostatic (which is activated by calorie deficits) and hedonic (which is activated by palatable foods). Our hedonic system drives us to eat more, even when we are full. Let's face it—you rarely eat a whole pint of ice cream because you are hungry. You eat it because it tastes delicious.

the leftovers at 1 a.m., or you just cannot resist another bowl of ice cream that is calling your name from the freezer. *If and when you do binge, the main thing to remember is to eat your next scheduled meal as if the binge never happened in order to get yourself back on track.* Everyone overeats sometimes—just don't let the binge sabotage your daily habits and start an unhealthy eating cycle. Even if you wake up the next morning feeling bloated and full, remember that it's a new day. Forget about the binge and eat a healthy breakfast so you don't get to lunch starving and ready to binge again.

Okay ladies, the workday is done and finally it is time to get to bed. Good thing the next chapter covers sleep. . . . I want to make sure you get the maximum benefit from your precious zzz's. . . .

PROFILE

Mrs. Smith, Esq., and Mr. Mom

Sarah was an attorney at a prestigious law firm. She was a litigator and took a lot of pride in winning tough cases. When she had a baby, she and her husband made a tough decision: Sarah would continue to work as the primary breadwinner while her husband would stay home and take care of their son, their home, the grocery shopping, and the cooking. While Sarah liked this setup (though she missed her son during the day), her main grievance was that her husband's cooking was making her fat! He did not feel like they had eaten a real meal unless there was some sort of beef on the table, and he would go between cooking huge, rich feasts and heating up unhealthy frozen dinners or, worse yet, full-fat mac and cheese. And because he indulged their son in whatever junk foods he wanted, there were always cookies, chips, soda, and ice cream tempting Sarah's sweet tooth when she finally got to sit down and watch her shows on the DVR at 10 p.m.

THE SOLUTION

Sarah and I decided that it was time for her to put her negotiation and communication skills to work for her family. She decided to bring her husband, Brad, to our nutrition sessions. Together, the three of us made up a standard weekly grocery shopping list for their family and decided that they should take a trip to the market together on Sunday mornings before the workweek got hectic.

We also came up with some healthy, filling, and easy things to cook that everyone could enjoy. We typed up these recipes and saved them on Brad's computer in a "Dinner" folder so he would always have an array of options from which to choose. We also put together a short list of healthy frozen dinners that Brad could heat up in a pinch.

Regarding the junk food, we vetoed soda all together. It was no favor to their son to be able to drink soda every day. Sarah also made a pact with her husband and son that they could buy one sweet snack per week (one carton of ice cream or one package of Oreos), to be consumed over the course of the week.

Sarah reports that over time, and with our proactive work, her family has found a healthy balance. Since the recipes we came up with were so easy (and delicious), Brad rarely defaults to frozen meals and they have both lost their love handles. Now, when Brad does cook up a rich feast, Sarah is able to enjoy it to the fullest (who doesn't like homemade spaghetti and meatballs every now and then?). Their son enjoys soda at birthday parties and on pizza/movie nights with his friends, but he understands the difference between healthy foods and treats.

PART 5

Lifestyle

CHAPTER 13

Get Wellness Soon

SLEEP, SUPPLEMENTS, WATER, BEAUTY, and weigh-ins are critical lifestyle elements that complement good eating habits. Fine-tuning these A-list priorities will make you look and feel better and more attractive. This chapter is devoted to encouraging you to take only the right supplements, drink lots of water, practice nutrition habits that will enhance your natural beauty, weigh yourself without stress, and sleep more. Which leads us to Healthy Habit #9: Aim for 7 to 9 hours of sleep per night.

Sleep

A lot of busy women feel like there is simply not enough time for ample sleep, or that sleeping is a waste of precious time. Though you are tired throughout the workday, many of you feel guilty about squandering personal time in bed, especially if it means trading off time spent at the gym, time spent with friends and family, or your ability to get an early start to the workday. Guess what—not only will the proper amount of sleep lead to greater alertness and productivity, it is also associated with improved mental health and staying slim.

So, how much sleep do we need? Healthy Habit #9 is explicit—7 to 9 hours per night for maximum functioning capacity. Revel in a full night's sleep and *do not feel guilty.* Our society often makes us feel lazy if we are not constantly "on the go." While it is true that some people can function with less sleep than others, the majority of us need a full night's sleep. Instead of feeling guilty about going to bed earlier or sleeping in, feel proactive: You are doing something good for your body, your joints, your muscles, and your mind.

Adequate sleep is a pillar of weight loss. The sleep habits of more than 238,000 female nurses enrolled in the Nurses' Health Study were analyzed over the course of 16 years. The results were conclusive: Women who slept less than 7 hours per night weighed more than women who slept 7 or more hours. Specifically, women who slept an average of 5 hours per night weighed approximately 5.4 pounds more than those who slept at least 7 hours. And the women who got more sleep actually exercised more and—not a big surprise—had slightly higher metabolisms, so they could (and did) eat more without weight gain.[1]

Fatigue often triggers reckless eating and an increased desire to graze, even after you've consumed your calorie budget for the day. Interestingly, lack of sleep increases the release of appetite hormones and makes you feel hungrier. Ghrelin is a hormone that makes us feel hungry; lack of sleep is associated with elevated ghrelin levels and increased appetite. Leptin is a hormone that regulates our food intake, making us feel satiated and full—and you guessed it—lack of sleep is associated with decreased leptin levels.[2]

 **CHEW ON THIS!**

Over the last two decades, average sleep duration in the United States has declined by 1–2 hours.[3]

So why can't I fall asleep, even when I am (or should be) exhausted? Some of us get restless when we can't fall asleep, tossing and turning and becoming more and more fixated on the fact that we are awake. It is important to note that your body still gets some rest as you lie in the darkness. This fact alone can soothe your anxieties about being unable to fall asleep, and thus may help you nod off. Other people have trouble falling asleep because they are disturbed by heartburn or gastric reflux. If you lie down right after eating, it can be painful and difficult to fall asleep. So, if you are a late-night snacker, consider this a good reason to leave the refrigerator door closed after 9 p.m. If you have difficulty sleeping because you find yourself wide awake at bedtime, analyze your caffeine intake. Caffeine can linger in the body for up to 12 hours—so try not to drink coffee after lunch (and never after dinner) if you have trouble falling asleep.

If you have trouble waking up in the morning, try to establish a consistent sleep and wake cycle and morning and evening routines throughout the week. Make sure to set your alarm at the same time every morning so your body clock gets used to that time—as you know by now, habits matter. Also, if you like, try to set your alarm earlier than you have to be up so you have the ability to snooze a couple times (because we all know snoozing

 CHEW ON THIS!

Heartburn can make it difficult to sleep due to a burning sensation in your throat and a sour stomach. If you are prone to reflux, beware of these foods before bed: alcohol, caffeine, citrus, and vinegar (in salad dressing), spicy foods, and high-fat foods (like that cookie that left a grease stain on your napkin). And don't eat too much at one sitting. Try sucking on a peppermint Tums—these can be very soothing and may help lull you to sleep. Talk to your doctor if these nutritional strategies are not enough to calm your heartburn.

is a daily fix). Or, set your alarm at the time when you want to get up, but put it on the other side of the room so you have to get out of bed to turn it off.

If you are getting enough sleep, but still feel tired all the time, check in with your doctor. Women are prone to thyroid gland disorders that can lead to feelings of sluggishness. These are easy to test and treat, if need be. Your doctor might also suggest a simple blood test for anemia (low iron stores).

If you aren't able to get a full night's sleep, make up missed zzz's with a catnap. A good nap length is somewhere between 20 and 30 minutes. This will give you the restorative benefits of sleep without the fatigue that comes on with a long bout of deep sleep. Make sure to set an alarm; knowing you will wake up when necessary will allow you to relax and fall asleep. And, if you worry about feeling sleepy when you wake up, try drinking coffee *before* you lie down. A 2003 Japanese study found that you can alleviate grogginess by drinking coffee before a nap since caffeine takes about 30 minutes to kick in (just enough time for you to nap).[4] So drink your cup, take a snooze, and wake up, ultra energized for the rest of the day. Remember, naptime is not just for kids, and getting a full night's sleep is not just for lazy adults.

Supplements

I am shocked by the scale and impact of the supplement industry, especially given the dearth of evidence that most of these products provide real health benefits. Some of the young women who I've counseled have followed excessive and dangerous regimens before I intervened. It is not normal to ingest 20+ pills in a day when you are in generally good health. If you are taking any dietary supplements daily, please consult with your family doctor to make sure your regimen is safe.

There is some cause to be concerned about the safety of supplements. The FDA requires that manufacturers of vitamins, herbal pills, and other dietary supplements *test their own products'* ingredients—there is no overarching regulatory body ensuring that supplements are free of contamination and impurities. This means that even the most innocent-looking supplements you find at your local health store are unregulated, and may be unsafe. In fact, Consumer Lab LLC, an independent lab that tests ingredients found in common supplements, has discovered dangerous contaminants, such as lead, in some products.

While people take supplements for different reasons at different stages in their lives, as a rule, vitamin deficiency is rare in this country because our abundant food supply has been fortified and enriched (our government requires the addition of vitamins and minerals to packaged foods in order to prevent deficiencies), and because we tend to eat plenty (the majority of us actually overeat). So, we pretty much get what we need from food—and that is the way it should be. Further, our bodies not only store some vitamins but also regulate their absorption—so if your intake is low one day but higher the next, your body adjusts.

All said, if you want extra assurance that you're getting enough vitamins and minerals, I recommend that you take a once-daily multivitamin. In particular, if you are on a weight-loss diet and eating less food than usual, a multivitamin can be a good call. Here are some tips that will help you choose the vitamin that's right for you.

 CHEW ON THIS!

Check out www.ConsumerLab.com to learn about the safety of your favorite supplements. Be sure to look at the Recalls and Warnings section.

- **Multivitamin:** Look for a multivitamin at your drugstore with 100 percent daily value of most vitamins and minerals, but not more. Research shows that nutrient supplements are the safest in small quantities—a mega-vitamin is *not* better.[5] In fact, fat-soluble vitamins A, D, E, and K can build up in your system and cause toxic effects, while water-soluble vitamins C and the Bs simply become expensive pee. That's right—when your body has too much, these are excreted via urine.

- **Iron:** The iron component in multivitamins can upset some people's stomachs, so take your multi with food. If you find that you still feel queasy (or constipated), switch to one without supplemental iron, but make sure you get enough of this mineral from food sources. Remember, women need approximately 18 mg per day. Meat, chicken, fish, dried fruit, or any food cooked in iron cookware (such as tomato sauce) are good sources.

- **Calcium:** Though the goal should be to get your 1000-mg calcium requirement from food sources, because this mineral is so important for our bones, I recommend taking supplemental calcium for insurance. On top of your multivitamin, which should provide you with about 300 to 500 mg of calcium (about all they can fit into one pill because calcium is bulky), I suggest you also take a 500-mg calcium pill at a different time of day, possibly before bed. It is crucial to take your cal-

CHEW ON THIS!

Studies show that taking dietary supplements is a characteristic of women who lead generally healthy lifestyles with adequate nutritional intakes via food.[6] This suggests that these supplement users do not in fact need to take supplements to overcome nutrient deficiencies or for any reason other than peace of mind.

cium at different times over the course of the day because this mineral is dose-dependent—you can only absorb so much at one time (about 500 mg).

◆ **Vitamin D:** Make sure your calcium supplement also contains 500 mg of vitamin D. Vitamin D facilitates the absorption and use of calcium by your body, so it is a key part of this supplement (this is why milk, with natural calcium, is fortified with vitamin D). Vitamin D functions like a hormone, and our bodies naturally synthesize it via sun exposure. For fair-skinned women, 10 to 15 minutes of sunlight per day is enough to get your daily dose, while women with darker skin pigment need a little more exposure. Because we are so frightened of the sun these days (with good reason), many women apply sunblock daily or avoid the sun altogether—and thus do not get enough Vitamin D. I say, wear your sunblock and make sure to drink fortified milk and take a calcium/vitamin D supplement every day.

◆ **Prenatal:** If you are pregnant or planning on getting pregnant, consult your doctor about a prenatal vitamin—nutrients such as folate, calcium, and iron are very important during pregnancy. For women of childbearing age (like us), taking 400 to 600 mcg of supplemental folate daily *before conception* is crucial. You want to have folate in your system at the time of conception and in the weeks right after to prevent fetal brain and spinal cord defects. Also, folate is one of the only vitamins that is better absorbed by your body in supplement form than from food (folate is generally found in green, leafy veggies)—so supplemental folate is the best way to go.

◆ **Omega-3:** Omega-3 fatty acid supplements have become all the rage these days. However, I recommend that you get your omega-3s—which may prevent or alleviate some cancers, heart disease, and arthritis—from food, not supplements.

Aim to meet Healthy Habit #7 and eat at least two servings of fish per week, sprinkle flaxseed on your cereal, grab a handful of walnuts for a snack, buy omega-3-fortified eggs, and cook with beans. Data is inconclusive about omega-3 supplements, which are typically either fish oil or algae based. They can be very expensive and may cause unpleasant side effects—among them, "fishy" burps. Further, you have to get fish oil supplements from a reputable source or they could be contaminated with the dreaded mercury or PCBs—these actually live in the fatty, oily part of the fish. The algae-based supplements have not been shown to have the same health-promoting benefits as the actual fish oil sources. Save your money and go for omega-3 foods.

◆ **Biotin:** A water-soluble B vitamin, biotin is an "in" supplement that many women take to promote hair and nail growth. Unfortunately, there is no research that has proven biotin to affect hair regrowth, but there are also no known adverse side effects and it is relatively inexpensive. So, while biotin should not harm you, the jury is still out on whether it is really worth taking. You can always eat foods that supply biotin if you are suspicious of supplements—almonds, milk, and strawberries all contain this vitamin.

◆ **Herbs:** I am not a big fan of herbal supplements for three reasons: (1) like vitamins, they are not regulated; (2) few reliable studies evidence the effectiveness or safety of supplemental herbs; and (3) some herbs can interfere with medications you may be taking as well as natural body systems (especially during pregnancy). Many herbal supplements also have a slew of potential side effects, and chief among them is GI distress. If you are interested in adding herbs to your diet, check with your doctor first.

Bottom line: Unless otherwise directed by your doctor, take a multivitamin and a calcium plus vitamin D supplement every day. Oh, and wash these pills down with a big glass of water . . . which leads me to our next topic . . .

Water

H_2O keeps our cells happy by preventing them from sticking together, and it plays a role in just about every single vital function of the body. Thirst is associated with feelings of confusion and sluggishness. Adequate hydration can be the cure-all for this brain fatigue, as the oxygen component of water gives us a natural boost of energy—without any calories or chemicals. The amount of water you need to drink for proper hydration varies depending on your activity level, size, sweat rate, and the climate in which you live. As a result, the Institute of Medicine has not set a specific daily goal for women. Instead, I advocate Healthy Habit #11: Drink water with every meal and throughout the day, every day. If you want a more specific goal to help you plan your water intake, make it a priority to gulp 8 to 12 glasses (8 ounces each) of delicious aqua every day.

In terms of what kind of drinking water is best, the answer is simple: Water from your tap should be just as clean as bottled water. This is because tap water typically goes through more screening and must meet higher safety standards than bottled

 CHEW ON THIS!

If you are worried about your municipal tap water, visit www. epa.gov/safewater to learn about your local drinking water quality.

water does. Tap water is regulated by the Environmental Protection Agency (EPA), whereas bottled is regulated by the U.S. Food and Drug Administration (FDA). Investing in a good-quality charcoal filtration system—either as an attachment to your sink tap or in a pitcher—is the safest way to go.

Incidentally, when you are on the go, drinking tap water in a reusable bottle is more environmentally friendly than buying bottled water. Think of all the glass and plastic used to make those disposable bottles—the manufacturing alone consumes a huge amount of petroleum. And full water bottles are heavy, which means a lot of oil is used in their transport. The "greenest" (and cheapest) option is to fill a dishwasher-safe, stainless steel water bottle (plastic bottles can harbor bacteria if they are not well cleaned) with filtered tap water every day.

While water should always be your first choice, you can consume any beverage to stay hydrated, including milk, juice, soda, and even coffee and tea (their diuretic role is often exaggerated). Also, many foods will help you meet your daily fluid needs—soup, fruit, vegetables, and dairy products are all more than 80 percent water. For example, a typical wedge of watermelon contains approximately 9 ounces (or more than a cup) of water.[7] Food also helps the body hold on to fluids because of the electrolytes it contains—minerals like sodium and potassium bind with water. Drinking beverages with meals and snacks will help you stay optimally hydrated.

Also, carbonated water is just as effective at hydrating the body as noncarbonated water. Carbonation is simply the addition of carbon dioxide to regular water. Unlike sugar, non-nutritive sweeteners, and caffeine, it has absolutely no effect on the nutritional quality of water, nor is carbonated water absorbed or metabolized differently than regular water. So drink 8 to 12 glasses of either flat or carbonated water—the choice is purely savory.

"Beautrition"

Good nutrition is as much about looking beautiful on the outside as it is about feeling good on the inside. What you put into your body dramatically affects three of our biggest beauty fixations: hair, skin, and the dreaded bloat. Forgo overpriced "miracle" creams and shampoos and wear your skinny jeans with confidence with these nutrition tips.

Radiant Skin

Skin is the body's largest organ and needs proper care and nourishment to look its best. For flawless skin:

◆ **Go for vitamin C.** A 2007 study of more than 4,000 women aged 40 to 74 found that high intake of dietary (not supplemental) vitamin C was associated with a lower risk of wrinkling and skin dryness, as well as better overall visual signs of aging.[8] Good news for those of you who love citrus. You can also purchase topical vitamin C products to be applied directly to your face at night before bed.

◆ **Eat an array of antioxidant-rich fruits and vegetables.** These will decrease free-radical damage to your skin and reduce formation of sunspots. Also—wear your sunblock every day (at least 30 SPF).

◆ **Try using vitamin E,** which protects against free-radical damage and will prevent and minimize wrinkles. You can buy vitamin E capsules, pierce them with a pin, and squeeze out the vitamin E to apply it topically.

◆ **Get your essential fats.** We need these to form healthy cells

Savvy Girl Tip

Because cosmetic vitamin C is very expensive, try saturating a cotton ball with lemon juice and wiping down your face with it before bed (be careful around your eyes). You will get the powerful antioxidant benefit without spending tons of moola.

and rejuvenate our skin. Yet another reason to enjoy olive oil and snack on walnuts.

- **Healthy Habit #9:** Aim for 7 to 9 hours of sleep per night. Sleep is a time for skin rejuvenation. Just make sure to keep your pillowcase clean. Change it *at least* once a week—bacteria and dust mites can cause breakouts.

- **Healthy Habit #11:** Drink plenty of water. Make sure to keep your skin well-hydrated. If you find yourself having to moisturize all the time, try increasing your water intake.

Shiny Hair

For most of us, our hair is integral to our self-image. If we aren't feeling confident, a "bad hair day" can easily turn into just a bad day overall. Here are some tips to properly feed your locks and keep them looking beautiful.

- **Eat plenty of low-glycemic-index foods,** such as whole grains, fruits, and veggies. A high-glycemic-index diet of processed, white carbohydrates like white bread and snack foods can lead to high insulin levels and a change in your hormones. This has been shown to cause male pattern baldness in women.

- **Go for those flavonoid antioxidants.** These can protect your hair follicles and encourage hair growth. Remember, coffee is a main source of antioxidants for many women—so get your daily fix and look good doing it.

- **Make sure to eat your omega-3 essential fatty acids.** They can improve hair texture by preventing your locks from becoming dry or brittle. Eat salmon and flaxseed to make your hair shine.

Bloat Reduction

All women complain about feeling bloated (not to be confused with fat) at least some of the time. Bloating can occur in your abdomen, but is also a common cause of puffy eyes, swollen feet, and chubby fingers. Deflate with these nutritional solutions:

◆ **Drink ample water and eat plenty of fiber.** *Together* these will keep your colon clean and rid your body of toxins.

◆ **Beware of wheat, which can sometimes cause bloating.** If you notice a sensitivity, try eating other whole grains like barley, millet, and oats and tell your doctor. She may want to test you for celiac sprue.

◆ **Aim to keep your sodium intake low.** This means the less processed food, the better. Sodium makes our body hold on to water, as does MSG, which should be avoided at all costs.

Weighing In on the Scale

Is facing the scale a healthy habit or an obsession? For some of you, the dreaded scale is collecting dust under your bed. For others, the number on the scale can control your mood and the outcome of your day. My recommendation is to weigh in one morning per week (the same day of the week) before breakfast, nude if possible, and always on the same scale. People naturally fluctuate within about 5 pounds over the course of a day due to water weight and hormone changes, so weighing yourself every day will not depict true weight change—it will really just display body water change (and can cause neurotic tendencies to kick in if the scale is slightly high). Furthermore, your morning weight is most accurate, because drinking just 16 ounces of fluid can tip the scale by 1 whole pound. The scale should not be something to fear. Consider it health maintenance, a way to keep yourself in check on a weekly basis so that extra pounds don't creep up on you.

Speaking of those extra pounds . . . it's time to hit the gym.

PROFILE

Underemployed and Oversupplemented

Olivia was unemployed, or as she liked to say, "in between jobs." Having time on her hands, she became obsessed with the only thing she could control—her food intake. She scheduled her whole day around what to eat for breakfast, lunch, and dinner (oh, and of course the occasional job interview). And, in her free time, she became supplement-happy, obsessively reading about them online, and visiting her local vitamin store daily to peruse the shelves. The problem was, in her quest to become the healthiest unemployed person around, she also became a thoroughly confused supplement junkie, ingesting upwards of 20 pills every day. While she bragged to all her friends that she was full of energy and would probably live forever on her new vitamin/mineral regimen, she also suspected that many supplements were probably excessive.

THE SOLUTION

I found Olivia's supplement regimen to be particularly troubling since she was a young, healthy woman who ate a balanced diet. We went through her daily pill routine and I urged her to get rid of all but the calcium supplement and to switch from a mega multivitamin to one with 100 percent or less of all vitamins and minerals—I recommended the One A Day Women's. Recently I got an e-mail from Olivia, who reported that she was feeling great, and without taking 20 supplements, was actually less constipated. What she was really surprised by, though, was how much extra money was left in her bank account at the end of the month. Her 20-pill regimen had been costing upwards of $200 per month. Now she spends that cash on weekly tennis lessons.

CHAPTER 14

Exercise: The Best Fix

INCORPORATING EXERCISE into your busy daily routine is key to health and weight management. That's why Healthy Habit #10 is twofold: Walk at least 30 minutes almost every day *and* work out 4 to 5 times a week at a higher intensity for at least 20 minutes. Most of my clients know that they need more exercise in their daily routine, but struggle to make it happen. My advice for them—and you—is to plan for exercise as if it were a mandatory meeting on your schedule, 4 to 5 days a week. This means you have to opt out if something comes up, instead of opting in if you happen to have time. When working out is a built-in component of your day, you are more likely to do it and you'll feel guilty if you skip out on a gym session. Otherwise, it can be tough to get motivated, and we all know how easy it is to make an excuse for avoiding it when you're busy. We working women are schedulers by nature, so use your planning skills to fit exercise in 4 to 5 times a week.

Why Exercise?

Exercise is perhaps the most important daily lifestyle fix. It is a fundamental habit for your long-term health that can help prevent heart disease, increase HDL cholesterol levels, lower blood pressure, and mitigate diabetes, some cancers, Alzheimer's disease, and insomnia. Furthermore, while calorie control and good nutrition are crucial for weight loss, exercise is an essential tool for weight management that helps promote increased bone mass. Exercise can also help change your body composition by replacing fat mass with muscle mass. This will actually raise your resting metabolism; a pound of muscle burns 35 to 75 calories per day while a pound of fat burns only about 2 calories per day.

Hitting the gym also benefits your mental health. In fact, exercise has been linked to reduction of depression,[1] and possibly the release of endorphins, the "happy" hormones like those released when we eat chocolate or have sex. You'll get the same mood-boosting benefits from your yoga class—without the extra calories (or the need for contraception). Studies have also shown that exercise helps to maintain and improve brain function, including response speed and working memory.[2]

Even if you are thin, you should aim to meet Healthy Habit #10. Slim but sedentary people can be "fat" on the inside. Maintaining your weight through diet alone can result in internal deposits of fat around the vital organs and put you at a higher risk for disease compared to overweight but active folks. A recent study of "thin" women conducted in the UK confirms this.[3] Of the hundreds of women tested, as many as 45 percent of those with a normal BMI (body mass index) had excess levels of internal (visceral) fat. There

CHEW ON THIS!

A 2005 study found that lean people tend to spend approximately two more hours per day standing, pacing, walking, or fidgeting than heavy people. More natural movement can actually mean a difference of up to 350 calories per day.[4]

is a big difference between just being thin and being healthy—and as a nutritionist, I want you to be both. The good news is that you can get rid of internal fat with regular exercise. So if you're not physically active already, today is the day to start.

Walking

The first part of Healthy Habit #10 stresses the importance of walking at least 30 minutes on most days of the week. The benefits of walking are often disregarded. For one thing, walking is accessible, free, and it is the most environmentally sound form of transportation around. Further, it is great for your heart, your waistline, and helps clear your head. It counts as "weight-bearing exercise" (you are bearing your own weight), and so is good for your bones, and it is low-impact, so it's easy on your joints. And with cell phones, BlackBerries, and iPods, a stroll does not have to be dead time. Here are some strategies to build walking into your busy life.

◆ **Walk to and/or from work.** My clients in New York City often tell me that they think about walking to work, but decide against it because they don't want blisters or shin splints from their heels or to be a sweaty mess when they arrive at work. I hear you—but I am also here to tell you that *using built-in, habitual lifestyle activities, such as a daily walk to work, can be a crucial way to maintain your weight, or to keep off lost weight.* So, take advantage of this daily time—especially if you live in a walking city, for goodness' sake. Try walking to and/or from work, or at least part of the way. If you want, get off the bus or subway early and walk the last 15 minutes each way. And, while it may be a fashion faux pas, wear comfortable sneakers and carry your dress shoes in your bag. It's also a good idea to keep a "refresher kit" in your desk so you can freshen up once you get to work.

- **Once you are at work, use the stairs.** Unless they are just too creepy to handle, there is no reason to take an elevator when you are only going up or down a couple of flights. Or, you can always get off the elevator a few floors early and walk the rest of the way—I'm not advocating that you walk up 30 flights each day.

- **Walk during your lunch hour.** Pick up your lunch, meet a lunch date out, or take a 15-minute breather and walk around the block and then go back to eat at your desk.

- **Don't let driving be the default.** If you are busy with errands on the weekend, put on your sneakers and iPod and get going. Even if you live in the 'burbs, walk up to 30 minutes, and don't drive to the local grocery store, dry cleaners, or drugstore. If you are going to be gone for a while, make sure to bring along a snack, like a small bag of almonds, so you are not trapped by the Starbucks Cookie Effect. Train yourself to walk when you would normally drive and only get in the car if you must.

- **Walk everywhere.** To the movies, out to dinner, to your friend's house, to church or synagogue, or anywhere else you like to go.

- **Use housework as exercise.** Vacuuming and laundry are both good ways to release energy and get in some movement.

- **Take a power walk.** Of course, whenever you can, take a 30-minute (or longer) power walk. It is my favorite source of exercise and can be a great time to catch up with a walking buddy or on the cell phone with your mom.

- **Note—if you would rather ride your bike than walk, go right ahead.** Just make sure to do it for about 30 minutes most days.

While 30 minutes a day most days may sound like a lot of time, you can usually get in at least two 15- minute walks if you decide to forgo a ride or public transportation and instead take a stroll in the fresh air—doesn't it sound sort of nice? You might even try using a pedometer to track your steps throughout the day, so you can see that every little bit counts. You may be surprised by the difference between a sedentary day and one that includes at least a 30-minute walk: a whopping 10,000 steps.

Higher-Intensity Exercise

Now, let's move on to the second part of Healthy Habit #10, or the goal of working out 4 to 5 times per week more vigorously, to get your heart rate up, tone your body, and sweat away the woes of the day. I have heard every excuse in the book from my clients for not working out—though usually, it boils down to one or more of the following issues: lack of time, lack of money, lack of motivation, or boredom. Here is what I have to say about these (lame) excuses:

Lack of Time

The workday holds distinct opportunities to work out: the morning before work, during your lunch hour, directly after work, or after dinner but before you go to bed. Try all four of these options to see which work best for you. Switch it up if you must to fit 4 to 5 days of exercise into your weekly schedule. And if you can only spare 20 minutes, that's fine. Just ramp up the intensity to get the most out of the time you have. There is no universal best time to work out—fit it in when you can and when you feel the best.

Note, when you work out first thing in the morning, you will burn more fat if you skip eating before your workout. As we know, your overnight fast puts you in starvation mode. Hitting the gym first thing brings your body farther into that state so it will rely on fat for fuel. The downside of this is that you will perceive your workout to be more difficult than it actually is since our muscles prefer to use carbohydrate when exercising. I advocate grabbing a high-carbohydrate snack before your workout (discussed on page 174). Also, some people may experience disturbances in sleep when working out at night (after dinner), while others may sleep better. Practice what feels right to you.

Lack of Money

There are many ways to work out for free (or nearly free). Try walking or running outside, try a yoga or workout video at home, or take advantage of your company's resources—they may be able to hook you up in all sorts of ways (discussed on page 171). Further, when you do spend money on a gym, trainer, lessons, etc., you are typically forgoing other activities like drinking, eating, or going to the movies that would cost money anyway. And don't worry about buying fancy workout clothes—instead, pick up some cute tanks at Target or Urban Outfitters. Just don't skimp on your sports bra (and double up if you need to) or workout sneakers.

Lack of Motivation

If being healthy and thin and feeling more energetic are not reason enough, here are some great motivators to get you moving:

◆ You want to look good for a specific event like your birthday party, a friend's wedding, a holiday soiree, or a date.

◆ Pick an activity you've always wanted to try and ask for it as a birthday or holiday gift. A new bike, a tennis racket, running sneakers, or sessions with a personal trainer are all great presents.

◆ Plan a vacation based on physical activity—like a ski trip to Vermont, a golf vacation in South Carolina, a bike tour of Napa Valley, or a hike on the Appalachian Trail. Before the trip, you will be pumped to train for the challenge.

- Train for a road race (biking or running). These are not as intimidating as you might think; many folks do them just to complete, not to compete.

- Spend an hour of your free time making a great workout mix that will pump you up at the gym all week long. Music can help you work out longer and at a higher intensity, so it can be a powerful tool to burn maximum calories and shrink your waistline.

Boredom

It's easy to get into a fitness rut. Listed here are some strategies to keep you from getting bored with any one activity. Mix it up a little and have fun with your workout.

- **Take a class at your gym**—when you find one you like that fits into your schedule, make it a habit and go once a week. Spinning, kickboxing, and Pilates are all good options that will help the time at the gym fly by.

- **Try yoga**—find a weekly class and a teacher you like, and schedule it in. Ashtanga, bikram, Baptiste, and power yoga are the most physically demanding yoga classes, so you may want to start in beginner classes (try easy hatha) and work your way up if you are new to yoga. Ask the studio to recommend the right class for you.

- **Work out with a friend**—this is one of the very best strategies because not only will you be letting yourself down if you bail, but you will be letting down your friend.

- **Take lessons**—try golf, squash, tennis, dance, and even running—another way to avoid excusing yourself from activity and you get to improve your skills or learn something wholly new. Then, translate these lessons into a weekly game/match/habit with a friend.

- **Include physical activity in your social plans**—every week meet for a power walk with your girlfriend or play a game of tennis or basketball with your boyfriend.

- **Join an adult sports league**—try basketball, baseball, or softball, coed football, volleyball, soccer, lacrosse, etc. If you were an athlete in college, this is a great way to keep up your game, be social and meet new people, and get some exercise doing what you love.

- **Swim**—this is a great calorie-burner and it is especially good for people with bad knees, joints, or plantar fasciitis. Join a gym with a pool, or check out your local YMCA, JCC, or the facilities at local high schools and colleges—they often have swimming hours open to the public.

- **Take advantage of your company's resources**—such as an onsite gym, reimbursement programs, health seminars, company-sponsored sports teams, free yoga or Pilates classes, or walking clubs or running teams. Talk to your HR department about all of these options—it can't hurt to ask, and you never know what you can get.

The strategies suggested above offer a plethora of options that include stretching, weight training, and aerobic exercise. While it is always a good thing just to get to the gym, it is best to do different workouts every day to work different muscle groups for optimal body toning (not to mention, to keep it interesting). Try multiple forms of physical activity by choosing two to five things that work for you. Make sure you are lifting weights (weight-bearing exercise is key for women to build bone and prevent osteoporosis); try interval or circuit training (it is the key to burning optimal calories); do aerobic exercise (it is great for your heart); and make sure to stretch (it is crucial for your muscles, posture, preventing/treating arthritis, and for other aches and pains).

Exercise FAQs

I want to address some important questions I am often asked about exercise, and dispel some popular misconceptions. Here are the top FAQs I encounter as a nutritionist:

*Should I allow myself extra calories if
I am working out regularly?*

Just because you are exercising does not mean you can eat whatever you want. While exercise can make us feel hungrier, or at least as if we should be able to eat more, we often over-compensate by consuming too many calories. The Obesity Society recently published a study that followed more than 300 overweight women who were prescribed different amounts of exercise but told not to diet. After six months, and as anticipated, they found that women who averaged 73 minutes of physical activity a week lost about 3 pounds, and women who averaged 136 minutes lost just over 4. However, what they were not expecting was that the women who exercised the most, about 190 minutes a week, lost only about 3 pounds.[5] The most intense exercisers were therefore making up for their calorie burns by unconsciously increasing their calorie intake.

It does not take very much food to overcompensate for calories burned during exercise. Think about it this way—it takes about 30 minutes on the elliptical machine to burn one Luna bar worth of calories. So, the bottom line is this: Don't subtract the calories you burn working out from your daily calorie budget, and don't add more food to your daily intake just because you have worked out.

How do I know how many calories I've burned?

Don't trust the calorie counts on your favorite aerobic machines at the gym! Makers of this equipment want you to feel good about yourself (and keep using their machines), so they inflate the calorie burn rate. Further, it is very difficult for an exercise machine to tell you exactly how many calories you are burning, especially because most machines don't account for body fat versus muscle mass. If two people weigh the same, the one with more muscle will burn more calories than the person with more fat. I typically divide the estimate the machine gives me in half to get a vague idea of how many calories I have burned.

Should I drink sports drinks or water?

You should always be hydrated prior to working out. Observe the color of your urine—if it's pale (the color of straw), you are hydrated and you can stop drinking about an hour before exercise to allow your bladder to empty and avoid disrupting your workout. Then, drink water to quench your thirst throughout your workout. You don't need a sports drink unless you are working out for more than an hour or in excessive heat. At that point, you will need a source of electrolytes and some carbohydrate with your fluid. Try Gatorade's G2—it has the same quantity of electrolytes as regular Gatorade and half of the carbohydrates (and calories). Or, you can dilute full-calorie sports drinks with water (1 part sports drink to 1 part water).

What are some good power snacks I can grab before hitting the gym?

Ten minutes prior to working out, a good snack would be high in carbohydrates and low in fat and protein. Carbohydrates fuel your muscles to work out at a high intensity. Try some fruit, like melon, a banana, or an orange—all are high in potassium and deliver carbohydrate (energy) to your bloodstream quickly.

An hour before working out, you could have one of the snacks I recommend in Chapter 9 for your midafternoon fix. Or try a packet of instant oatmeal, a small container of fat-free yogurt, a 100-calorie Balance bar, or ½ cup cereal with skim milk. Also, go for your coffee fix. Caffeine can increase your alertness while working out so you can ramp up your intensity. A 12-ounce latte with soy milk is a great power snack to give you the caffeine boost and some carbohydrate from the milk.

Three hours prior to exercise, try to eat a meal similar to one of the lunch options in Chapter 8. This meal should include lean protein to keep you satisfied, and include that carbohydrate to keep your energy stores high. It should also be lower in fat. A high-fat meal (think fried food or regular ground beef) can take 9 to 12 hours to empty out of the stomach and may make you feel sick after working out. Go for turkey, canned salmon, or natural peanut butter on whole grain bread and a Greek-style yogurt on the side.

When and what should I eat after working out?

After working out, you have a 30- to 60-minute window to eat. If you wait longer, your body will go into starvation mode and you will not burn calories as efficiently. Also, if you wait too long, you will likely get overly hungry and may make a bad decision about what to eat. Use the plate method discussed in Chapter 11 to create a satisfying post-workout meal: Fill a quarter of your plate with lean protein, a quarter with starch, and half with veggies. If the recovery meal is breakfast, try 2 eggs, 2 pieces of whole grain toast, and ½ cup low-fat yogurt. After exercising, your body is trying to bring itself back to homeostasis and needs some protein and carbohydrate to do so.

How should I schedule my workouts?

While I encourage you to think critically about what exercise schedule will work best for you, I have found that a Monday through Thursday plus Saturday workout schedule, with Friday and Sunday off, works best for many of my clients. Again, think about the options you have for when to work out (a.m., lunch, afternoon, p.m., or weekends) to make your own schedule. Here is a sample:

M: walk 30 minutes / do yoga

T: walk 30 minutes / take a spin class

W: walk 30 minutes / go to the gym to do the elliptical machine and lift weights

Th: walk 30 minutes / play tennis with a friend

F: walk 30 minutes / off

Sa: walk 30 minutes / do a power walk with a friend

Su: walk 30 minutes / off

You are almost at peak health—eating well and working out regularly. But there are still a few lingering ailments that most of us know about all too well. I'll tackle those next.

ExerciseSlump.com

Jess worked at a start-up in Silicon Valley. She absolutely loved her job, not only because she liked the work, but also because she had hip and intelligent colleagues and her bosses were very cool; they actually cared about work/life balance and treated every employee with respect. Problem was, even with the right job and cool bosses, Jess could not find the time to work out during the week. Like so many of us, Jess couldn't bring herself to get out of bed one minute earlier to go to the gym in the morning, even though she knew this was probably the most practical time of the day for her to work out. At lunch, she was often plagued by guilt because there was a nice employee gym and shower downstairs at her office, but it just seemed too complicated to rush away from her desk, work out, re-shower, dress, and put on makeup in one hour. And besides, this was her main time of day to chill out a little and gossip with co-workers. At the end of the day, Jess was a victim of working late. She was supposed to work a 9 a.m. to 6 p.m. day, but often ended up staying at work till more like 7 or 8 p.m., and was just too tired and antsy to get home at that point to jet to the gym. Working was a full-time gig during the week for Jess, and exercise always took a back seat.

THE SOLUTION

Jess needed to concoct a weekly workout schedule. We discussed some strategies, and decided that her best plan of attack was to work other folks into her exercise regimen. For example, on Mondays, Jess could spend some of her hard-earned dough to meet with a personal trainer in the evening. Tuesday morning, she could plan a recurring yoga date with her best friend. Wednesday she could make a pact to gossip with her colleague while they worked out together at the office gym during lunch. Thursdays she could sign up to play in an evening adult sports league (she was a great lacrosse player in college). Jess could plan to take Friday off—to have a mellow lunch with other co-workers and a relaxing evening, and then Saturday morning she could have an ongoing date to meet her friend (and her friend's dog) for a long and chatty power walk.

Jess reports she is on target with working out these days. She is following through with her daily exercise plans because she can't let the others down. Also, Jess says that the variety in both activity and time slot makes each workout less tedious, more fun, and easier to commit to.

CHAPTER 15

Things We Don't Like to Discuss

THIS CHAPTER DEALS with a few of our least favorite things: constipation, irritable bowel syndrome (IBS), yeast infections, urinary tract infections (UTIs), premenstrual syndrome (PMS), polycystic ovary syndrome (PCOS), low libido, migraines, and stress. As you likely know, these ailments are common among women our age. Though we don't like to talk about most of them in polite company, all of these irritating issues can be improved, minimized, and possibly even eliminated through the nutritional strategies I'm about to share with you.

Gastrointestinal (GI) Disorders

Constipation

Though everyone has different "pooping norms"—some of us go twice a day and others only every other day—if you are having two or fewer dry bowel movements per week accompanied by feelings of bloating and straining, you are likely a bit clogged up. Though constipation is a very common disorder among women, and chief complaint among many of my clients, we don't like to talk about it. (My husband tries to convince himself that I do not poop or fart, as if these bodily functions are somehow limited to men.) So let's get over the fact that it is a little embarrassing (if you have been pregnant, you are likely already more evolved on the topic) and do something about it . . . quickly. We want to prevent hemorrhoids at all costs—constipation can cause swelling of the rectum veins and the formation of these painful pouches. If you think you have hemorrhoids already, consult your doctor and get on the constipation prevention bandwagon discussed here.

Savvy Girl Tip

If, despite your best efforts, you find yourself constipated, try eating a serving of dried fruit (prunes, apricots, dates, or raisins) accompanied by a large glass of water. This should help get things moving again. . . .

No matter when you begin to think about your bathroom break, having a "safe" place to go is key—and it isn't always the easiest feat at work, when your boss might be in the stall next to you. This can be one reason we end up feeling constipated. You must figure out a daily situation that is comfortable for you. Try to get on an early-morning or late-evening "poop schedule" so you can go in the privacy of your own home. The main rule of thumb, though, is that if you have to go—go. Holding it in only makes constipation worse.

Drinking plenty of water, eating enough fiber, and getting exercise are the key ingredients to keeping your digestive system regular. As mentioned earlier, aim for 25 to 35 grams of fiber per day from fruits and dried fruits, veggies, cereal grains, and whole grain breads, pastas, and rices. These will add the necessary bulk to your stool to push it along for elimination. But beware—eating too much fiber without enough water can be a deadly combo—you will end up bloated and uncomfortable.

Here I stress the importance of Healthy Habit #11: Drink water. Water is a crucial partner to fiber in the match against constipation. Check to make sure you are not dehydrated—if you are, your pee will be dark yellow instead of clear or very light. Also, don't wait until you are thirsty to drink—by the time you feel parched, you have probably already lost 2 or more cups of your total body water. Always have a full water bottle with you as you work, exercise, run errands, and especially when it is hot and you are enjoying time outside.

A lot of folks wonder if they should use Metamucil or other fiber supplements to ease constipation. Generally, I advocate eating the right foods over taking these unpalatable supplements, which can cause their own bloating and flatus. However, some conditions such as thyroid disease, pregnancy, or diabetes and some medications like antidepressants, narcotic pain meds, and iron supplements can cause chronic constipation. I urge you to talk to your doctor about your individual situation and she can help determine the best course of treatment. Otherwise, skip the supplements and go for wholesome foods, water, and plenty of physical activity.

So—now that we know how urine should look (clean and clear) and how poop shouldn't look (dried-out little plops), I want to share with you how your poop *should* look. A healthy colon (a.k.a. the large intestine or gut) will produce feces that are long

 **CHEW ON THIS!**

To prevent digestive distress, it's good to understand how your body processes food. The system works like this: FOOD → mouth → esophagus → stomach (food breakdown) → small intestines (food use via enzymes) → colon or large intestines (storage for excess fiber and waste) → rectum. Problems at any stage of this process will cause you to suffer the effects of heartburn, acid reflux, or indigestion.

and continuous, and possibly curved or C-shaped. This makes perfect sense because the colon, which is the final resting spot for our undigested foodstuffs before we eliminate it, is sort of an upside-down U in shape. So—if we have the proper bulk-to-liquid ratio, our feces should follow this path out of our bodies.

Irritable Bowel Syndrome (IBS)

Take the discomfort of constipation one step further, and you have IBS. It's important to discuss this uncomfortable situation because close to 20 percent of the adult population has Irritable Bowel Syndrome or IBS-like symptoms—it is a very common diagnosis.[1] IBS (a.k.a. spastic colon) typically afflicts women in their twenties, and stress, anxiety, and other lifestyle factors may play a role in its development. IBS is characterized by alternating constipation and diarrhea due to reduced motility in the lower digestive tract. Symptoms include abdominal cramping, bloating, gas, diarrhea, and sometimes, severe pain. Fatigue and headache may also trouble victims of IBS. Though it causes a great deal of discomfort, IBS does not damage your intestines or cause ensuing disease. It should not be confused with Inflammatory Bowel Disease or IBD, which includes the more serious Crohn's disease and ulcerative colitis. Consult with your doctor if you think you could be suffering from IBS, as medical treatment is available for severe cases. Listed here are some dietary provisions for dealing with IBS and its related symptoms.

- ◆ Healthy Habit #11—drink water. Hydration is key for IBS sufferers. Make sure to drink plenty of water (at least eight 8-ounce glasses per day) throughout the day for optimal digestive health.

- ◆ For IBS with diarrhea, eat foods high in soluble fiber. These will add bulk to your stool without digestive discomfort and will slow transit time. Try oatmeal, bananas, potatoes, legumes, or pears.

◆ For IBS with constipation, try insoluble fiber, which will increase transit time through the colon and so decrease heaviness in the colon. Eat whole grain foods, fruits (dried or fresh with skins), and veggies.

◆ Artificial sweeteners, fried or high-fat foods, dairy products, carbonation, alcohol, caffeine, and also decaffeinated coffee can exacerbate IBS—review your food journal and try to correlate your symptoms with any of these irritants.

◆ Gum-chewing can aggravate IBS by introducing air into your already bloated stomach. Try sipping ginger or mint tea after a meal instead—you can freshen your breath and soothe your stomach at the same time.

◆ Eating too quickly can exacerbate IBS—chew and swallow each bite thoroughly before digging in for a second bite.

◆ Try incorporating probiotics into your diet. These beneficial bacteria may reduce inflammation and help you maintain a healthy colon and digestive tract. Look for acidophilus or lactobacillus supplements with at least 10 billion colony-forming units per capsule. I suggest Culturelle, which you can google and order online. Take these with meals. Also, try eating a yogurt or cereal enhanced with probiotics every day.

Girly Infections

Yeast Infection

Or should we call them Yuck Infections. Nearly 75 percent of women will get at least one in her lifetime.[2] We know the common symptoms—vaginal burning and itching and abnormal discharge due to the overgrowth of yeast. Yeast actually lives in the vagina full-time, but due to an array of factors—tight, non-porous clothes, stress, lack of sleep, taking antibiotics or other medicines—it can proliferate and cause infection. You should call your doctor when you suspect that you have a yeast infection and she can write you a prescription for an antifungal cream or recommend an over-the-counter treatment.

You can also help treat or prevent a yeast infection through your diet. If you are prone to yeast infections, eat a plain yogurt containing acidophilus every day. You can also take the probiotic acidophilus supplements to fight a yeast infection (and soothe your IBS at the same time).

In addition, there are a few foods to avoid. It's best to eliminate refined sugars, fermented foods, and yeast products from your diet until inflammation subsides. These can cause an overgrowth of yeast in the intestinal tract and slow your recovery. So skip breads and other baked goods, aged cheeses, alcohol, caffeine, vinegar, pickles, and dried fruits. And remember, avoid tight clothing and wear cotton panties for a few days, and if you go swimming or to the gym, change out of your wet/sweaty clothes as soon as possible.

Urinary Tract Infection (UTI)

Also known as a bladder infection, a UTI occurs when bacteria attach to your urinary tract walls and travel to the bladder and sometimes the kidneys. Symptoms include frequent and painful urination, sometimes accompanied by blood.

Consult your doctor if you feel one coming on and immediately start chugging pure cranberry juice (not to be confused with sugar-infused cranberry juice cocktail). Cranberry is one of the best remedies for a bladder infection as it may contain a substance that keeps those wretched bacteria from attaching to your urinary tract walls and inhibits bacterial growth. You can also take cranberry capsules (available at most drugstores) with water. And speaking of water, flood your body with water to treat your UTI. The bladder cleanses itself each time you urinate. Drink at least an 8-ounce cup every hour to stay hydrated, dilute the bacteria, and make this dreaded affliction less painful. In addition, stay away from caffeine and alcohol, which have an adverse effect on the bladder and can be dehydrating. If the effects aren't mitigated, see your doctor right away. If left untreated, a UTI can spread to your kidneys and become very dangerous.

Common causes of UTIs include sexual intercourse, "holding it" when you have to urinate (which stretches the bladder and, over time, weakens it), and pregnancy. To prevent a UTI in the future, always urinate after intercourse to flush away any bacteria that enter during sex. Also, wear cotton, breathable undies and wipe from front to back when you go to the bathroom.

Hormonal Stuff

Premenstrual Syndrome (PMS)

Ranging from debilitating to only slightly annoying, PMS symptoms such as cramps, bloating, depression, fatigue, breast tenderness, anxiety, food cravings, and acne afflict the majority of women each month, typically a week before the onset of their period. There are different causes for these symptoms including fluctuating hormones (estrogen and progesterone), a reduction in the hormone serotonin, and unstable blood-sugar levels. The good news is, your diet can help to lessen the effects of PMS. Try some of these suggestions to get you through this unpleasant time of the month.

◆ Follow the Daily Fix regular meal and snack plan including fruits, vegetables, whole grains, and lean protein. It will keep your blood-sugar levels stable. Further, your metabolism slightly increases with menstruation—so make sure to satisfy your appetite with regular and consistent food intake.

◆ Follow the physical activity recommendations in Chapter 14. Exercising regulates your hormone levels and allows you to sweat out some of the ickiness you are likely experiencing.

◆ Eat extra whole grain foods like brown rice, whole wheat breads, and veggies. The fiber content can help remove excess estrogen and the starch content can curb your cravings for serotonin-boosting carbohydrates.

◆ To get rid of PMS bloat, do not salt your foods and go for naturally low-salt whole foods. Stay away from high-salt processed foods like soups, lunch meats, bacon, cheese, and chips.

◆ Healthy Habit #11—Drink tons of water (and green tea as well) to dilute you body's water-to-salt ratio. Although it may sound counterintuitive, drinking more water decreases bloating by diluting your salt content. Try for at least one 8-ounce glass per hour.

◆ Take calcium supplements daily, starting a week before your period. Studies have shown that calcium can reduce PMS symptoms by as much as 30 percent.[3]

◆ Try a supplement with magnesium if you are feeling constipated—it can help relieve some of the pressure and bloating.

◆ Because you lose iron with your period, this is a good time of the month to enjoy a steak (just make sure it is not bathed in salt), as well as other iron-rich foods like beans and legumes, other lean proteins like fish and chicken, and dried fruits.

Polycystic Ovary Syndrome (PCOS)

Genetic factors cause a predisposition to PCOS, a hormonal imbalance that is thought to affect 5 to 10 percent of females in the reproductive age group.[4] Irregular menstrual periods, possible fertility problems, and ovarian cysts characterize PCOS. A slightly high level of male hormones can also cause PCOS sufferers to have acne, facial hair growth, and male pattern hair loss. Those afflicted often crave junk food and frequently become overweight or obese, leading to insulin resistance and type 2 diabetes. If you think you suffer from PCOS, consult with your doctor right away. The first line of defense against this condition is weight loss via a balanced diet, regular exercise, and Healthy Habit #11—ample water intake. Make sure to follow the Daily Fix plan. Shedding excess weight or preventing weight gain is literally the key to living harmoniously with this condition.

Low Libido

When you experience low libido, not only do you crave less sex, but you often feel less sexy. In terms of nutrition, diets very low in fat can leave women with low estrogen and testosterone levels. Your body needs fat to make these hormones for sexual response and ample lubrication. Further, chronic dieting is stressful and energy-sapping in and of itself, and therefore can affect your sex drive. Don't be afraid of fat, and make sure you are getting about 25 to 30 percent of your daily calories from it. Of course, you should always choose the good, heart-healthy unsaturated varieties found in foods like almonds, avocados, and olive oil. Also, Healthy Habit #11 helps protect your sex drive because hydration is absolutely key to reducing vaginal dryness, which can make any sexual activity mighty uncomfortable.

If you're experiencing diminished libido and your fat and water intake seem to be appropriate, check with your doctor. If you are take a birth control pill, you may need to switch to a brand with a different hormone level. Low thyroid function, anemia, low-level depression, or use of other medications can also affect sex drive.

And since we are on the subject of libido and food, why not try some of our favorite aphrodisiacs—oysters, chocolate, honey, strawberries, and mangoes, to name a few? In reality there is little to no science to "aphrodisiac food" but they can have a placebo effect whereby you believe that they will enhance your sex drive—and thus, put you in the mood.

Migraine

These severe headaches, often accompanied by nausea and visual disturbances, afflict more women than men.[5] A number of things can trigger a migraine headache, including constipation, stress, weather, lack of sleep, hormonal changes, or a genetic predisposition to the condition. When you feel a migraine coming on, drink a cup of strong coffee or take a migraine-specific pain reliever that contains caffeine immediately and lie down in a dark, quiet room. Sometimes this will nip a migraine in the bud, but if the symptoms persist (these headaches can linger for days), you should call your doctor. You may need prescription medicine to alleviate your headaches. Recently, antidepressants have also been found to be an effective treatment for some migraine sufferers. Your headache may be triggered by a low serotonin level—which can also cause depression—and so drugs targeting this hormone may be an effective treatment for migraine.

In order to prevent a migraine from erupting or to function through the haze, eat small meals and snacks through the day to prevent blood-sugar swings. Get some light exercise if you can— even walking in the fresh air can be soothing, depending on the severity of your headache. Make sure to eat high-fiber foods and follow Healthy Habit #11—drink water. Avoid alcohol (especially red wine, which is high in tannins), cigarettes, MSG (in Chinese food) and nitrates (preservatives in lunch meat and hot dogs), all of which are common migraine triggers.

Stress

Unfortunately, we career-driven ladies are no strangers to stress. Stress is your body's response to a demand or situation that makes you feel frustrated, angry, or anxious. Extensive research has been conducted on the association between stress and weight gain, and on the hormone cortisol, which may be released in response to stress and can cause abdominal weight gain. But studies to date are overwhelmingly inconclusive, despite the plethora of full-page magazine advertisements touting this connection. However, in 2007, researchers at Georgetown University identified a neurochemical pathway that promotes fat accumulation in the bellies of stressed mice when coupled with access to unlimited food.[6] This research may suggest a link between chronic stress, much like that which we experience in the American workplace, and our obesity epidemic.

Moreover, in 2008, the American Dietetic Association published a study of more than 800 subjects aged 18 to 83 who were given a questionnaire regarding emotional and stress-related

 CHEW ON THIS!

A 15-minute weekly massage is associated with reduced psychological stress and anxiety, increased immune function, and improved sleep. For busy women, a weekly relaxation ritual that is both soothing and therapeutic, but also quick and affordable, makes for a practical boost you should not resist.[7]

eating. Individuals who reported to be the most stressed were thirteen times (!!!) more likely to be overweight or obese compared with those who experienced little stress.[8] Eating is obviously a coping mechanism to alleviate stress.

Whether you gain weight when you feel stressed, or lose your appetite due to anxiety, it is simply undesirable to go through life struggling with the burden of stress. While we cannot completely eradicate it from our lives, I urge you to combat it proactively by starting a weekly—if not daily—relaxation ritual. I recommend any of the following:

◆ Try yoga, Pilates, meditation, and deep breathing

◆ Get your blood flowing with exercise of any type

◆ Give yourself a beauty treat—massage, facial, mani, pedi

◆ Take a catnap once a week—research shows that sleep decreases stress hormones

◆ Take a bath with relaxing salts or bubbles

◆ Read—put yourself in a different world to relax your mind

◆ Watch a movie one night a week

◆ Get together with your girl group, chat it up, and vent— research shows that companionship with girlfriends can alleviate stress through sharing stories and commiserating—just watch what you eat and drink!

Okay, I hope by now you're feeling better, because it looks like you are going on a business trip in our next and final chapter. . . .

PROFILE

Sh*t Doesn't Happen

Emerson was a ninth grade English teacher and high school field hockey coach. She believed in hard work (both in the classroom and on the field) and only gave out A's if her students handed in near-perfect work. She felt that her students generally respected her, but also suspected that they whispered behind her back. In fact, one time she heard two girls gossiping about how "uptight" and "by-the-book" she was. When Emerson came to me, she desperately wanted to loosen up a little—and in more ways than one. She had been suffering from terrible constipation.

THE SOLUTION

Clearly, it was no fun to walk around feeling constipated and bloated. We went over different tactics to combat Emerson's dirty little secret. First and foremost, Emerson needed to up her intake of water. Today she aims to drink at least eight 8-ounce glasses every day and sends herself reminders to drink water every hour via her BlackBerry. Next, Emerson needed to eat more fiber. Now, she starts her day with Fiber One or Kashi cereal with skim milk and a piece of fruit, and eats additional fruit, vegetables, and whole grains galore through the day. Finally, Emerson needed more exercise to get her bowels moving. Now she is playing field hockey with her athletes instead of just coaching from the sidelines. She feels so much better now that she has dealt with her sh*t (okay, pun intended).

CHAPTER 16

Travel Traps

AHH—THE JOYS of business travel. It is a basic require-ment for many jobs, but can pose a major challenge to our waistlines. Traveling separates us from our routines, as well as from our standard food and physical activity resources. Fur-ther, your schedule is often not your own, and time is typically of the essence, packed with meetings, deadlines, and manda-tory social events. *The Daily Fix* has already equipped you with a slew of good habits for the workday, as well as the nec-essary tools to combat the trickiest meal and snack scenarios. First and foremost, I urge you to do your best to follow our plan while traveling for business. Now I'll unveil Healthy Habit #12: A workday is a workday, regardless of where you are. Learn to practice *The Daily Fix* while traveling for busi-ness and proceed with your healthy meal/snack/ physical activ-ity choices. You have my sympathies—this is not always going to be easy. Here are some specific travel traps and strategies to combat them.

Healthy Habits for Business Travel

Trap: Packing

While frantically packing the night before a business trip, you decide at the last minute not to bring your gym clothes because your sneakers just take up too much room in your luggage and conflict with your eternal quest to pack only a carry-on.

Fixes:

◆ No matter what, bring your workout clothes. Don't sacrifice your health just so you don't have to check bags. Besides, with a bigger suitcase, you can also bring your own hair dryer and forgo the one that never really works in the hotel.

◆ Wear your sneakers on the plane if packing space is tight. They are the best choice for running from one gate to another anyway.

◆ Call ahead to see if your hotel has a lap pool. Then bring your suit and goggles—these take up minimal packing space and swimming can be the most refreshing way to wake yourself up after a long, jetlagged sleep.

Trap: The Plane

Many business trips start at the airport, where unfortunately, healthy food is scarce. You often arrive after a tough commute,

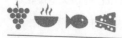

CHEW ON THIS!

Researchers have discovered that when we consistently practice a habit, we create new synaptic pathways in our brains and even form new brain cells if the process is repeated frequently enough. By following your Healthy Habits, you can literally rewire your brain for health![1]

feeling exhausted and famished. It's tough to battle the temptations all around—Cinnabon smells wafting through the air can sabotage the willpower of any innocent-but-hungry bystander.

Fixes:

◆ Eat before you even get to the airport. Starting your trip at home with a square, healthy meal is the best way to nip a potential calorie barrage in the bud. If you are unable to eat at home before your flight, airports usually do offer yogurt, fruit, energy bars, and sandwiches. Your best option is likely a Subway 6-inch sandwich or the above snacks from a refrigerated case at the newsstand or coffee shop, along with a coffee or tea.

◆ While you are on the plane, don't let down your guard and eat a bag of potato chips, a prepackaged cookie (half-frozen), and crackers with high-fat, spreadable cheese. Pack your own food in your shoulder bag and skip this airplane fare altogether. Have a ready-to-eat snack, such as an energy bar, a bag of nuts and/or dried fruits, a bag of high-fiber cereal, fresh fruit or veggies, whole wheat crackers and low-fat cheese, or a sandwich or salad. Review all of our meal and snack options covered in *The Daily Fix* to see what makes the most sense to pack up for your trip.

◆ Every time a beverage is offered, go for bottled water and skip the alcohol that will dehydrate you or the carbonated sodas that can cause bloating. As important as water is for general daily consumption, it is even more crucial in helping you stay hydrated when you travel. In-flight air is extremely drying and is literally akin to being in the desert at near-zero humidity. Make sure to drink only bottled water on the plane and stay away from the ice cubes (airplane tap water is known to be recycled). Try to buy a big bottle once you are through security so you don't have to bug your stewardess every five minutes.

◆ Get up and walk around routinely while you are flying—try to walk up and down the aisle at least once every hour. And choose an aisle seat whenever you can so you don't have to worry about climbing over the person next to you every time you get up.

◆ Stretch out your arms and legs before you sit back down and while you are sitting, try to "write the alphabet" out with your feet as a way to activate and stretch your ankles and calves.

Trap: **The Hotel**

After a long trip, you are bound to feel out of sorts. You have likely been sitting in a cramped seat with dry air all around you, and chances are, you are unfamiliar with your new surroundings.

Fixes:

◆ After checking into your hotel, it's tempting to just crash for the night and order room service. But the very best thing you can do (before unpacking or rushing off to a meeting) is to take a quick walk or hit the hotel gym. Getting your circulation going and stretching are both key to feeling rejuvenated after an airplane ride. Then take a quick shower and settle into your trip feeling refreshed.

◆ Try to stay in a hotel with a fitness center and/or a lap pool. Check online for these amenities before booking your stay, or request that your corporate travel agent do the same.

◆ Walk whenever you can instead of jumping in a cab. In addition to getting in some exercise, you'll also get to explore a new city.

◆ Go for a run to get to know your new surroundings. Ask your concierge about the safety of the area, and inquire about a jogging map or even a running guide/partner—many hotels offer these services.

◆ Get to bed at a reasonable hour. It is crucial to get enough zzz's, especially since you may already be a little run-down from exposure to germs on the plane or lost hours due to time zone differences. It's a lot easier to wake up early the next morning and get on the treadmill if you have had enough sleep.

Savvy Girl Tip

If you get traveler's diarrhea, remember to be a BRAT. That is—try the BRAT diet of bland, easy-to-digest fare: Bananas, Rice, Applesauce, Toast/Tea.

◆ Try to work out in the morning, before the jam-packed workday starts. Or, if your meetings begin too early, try to get in a 30-minute workout at the end of the day, before dinner, to energize you for the rest of the evening (it can be more invigorating than a nap).

◆ If you have only twenty minutes to call and check in at home, go for a walk while you talk on your cell phone.

◆ Whenever you can, use the stairs instead of escalators or elevators.

◆ Ask the hotel to remove your minibar or have it locked up. Let's face it—the offerings are mostly overpriced junk foods.

◆ When ordering room service, follow our Daily Fix strategies—you know how to navigate a menu at this point. Also, look for "healthy" designations to help you make your selections.

◆ If there is a spa in your hotel and you have time, rejuvenate with a massage or even just with a dip in the hot tub. Loosening up your muscles after traveling is never a bad idea.

Trap: **Food**

Too often we use travel as an excuse to eat poorly and end up feeling constipated and bloated. Salt overload from processed and restaurant food and lack of healthy, high-fiber options can take a toll on your system.

Fixes:

◆ Your strategy should be to choose foods that are more or less akin to what you would eat at home during the workweek. Remember, this is business travel, not spring break.

◆ Whenever you can, make it a priority to eat high-fiber foods and drink ample amounts of water with and between each meal to keep your GI system on track.

◆ As always, start your day with a healthy breakfast, try a salad for lunch (follow our salad guide), and make sure to follow our tips for dining out. Take advantage of www.MenuPages.com, a guide to restaurant menus across the country, to get an idea of dinner offerings so you can plan out your healthy meal.

◆ If you are going to another country or somewhere very exotic, bring a jar of peanut butter, a couple of cans of water-packed tuna, and some energy bars in your luggage just in case you are unable to find an appealing square meal.

◆ Have a sick stomach kit, complete with an antacid like Tums for heartburn, a stool softener like Colace for constipation, and an antidiarrheal like Immodium for you-know-what.

What about Leisure Travel?

Unlike travel for work, during which I urge you to follow the Daily Fix eating plan, while you are on vacation, I want you to just enjoy yourself. The crux of my book is that your workday, typical, routine habits should be clean so you can splurge a little on special occasions. So, as they say, when in Rome . . . if you are camping, eat s'mores; if you are in Paris, enjoy a croissant; and when in Rome—eat pizza!!

A really good way to go about a week's vacation is to alternate every other day between health and pure decadence—this way you will truly feel like you have gotten the full indulgent experience that a vacation should offer, but you will not feel like a glutton who has overdone it. Or else indulge in the cuisine every day, but continue to exercise as frequently as is possible and enjoyable. Trust me, it will make the delicacies taste even better.

You are finally equipped with a total plan to eat cleanly during your hours at work—wherever that may be—so you can enjoy the true indulgences in life, such as a vacation with your best friend or hubby.

PROFILE
Business Trips? Just Watch the Chips

Casey was a consultant for a prestigious management-consulting firm in Boston. After graduating from business school, she was thrilled to accept this coveted position. Her only grievance was the amount of travel her job required. She typically spent three or four of her weekdays at the client's offices, which were often scattered throughout the country. While Casey loved her projects, it was hard for her to feel healthy when her schedule was so erratic, she was living out of a suitcase, and she ate the majority of her meals at the airport, in a conference room, at a client dinner, or via room service.

THE SOLUTION

Because Casey's work revolved around travel and change, she needed to build healthy habits into each day and practice them no matter where she was. More specifically, Casey and I identified some common travel-related calorie traps and came up with strategies to combat them.

To begin, Casey planned ahead for travel days by preparing and packing ready-to-eat meals and snacks. She also pledged to buy a large bottle of water each time she finished getting through security at the airport. I advised her to start the workday with a healthy breakfast, whether it was in a hotel room, conference room, or restaurant. The goal was to aim for either high-fiber cereal with skim milk and fruit, or egg whites with whole wheat toast and fruit. These breakfasts were easily available and would ensure that Casey started the day with the right kind of energy to sustain her through the morning. In meetings, Casey pledged to pass up the standard spread of cookies and brownies and to instead sip on the hot coffee and teas and snack on the fruit. When she went out to extravagant client dinners, Casey kept within her daily calorie budget by employing strategies such as ordering two appetizers, or leaving half of her entrée on the plate. She also took advantage of her hotel's fitness center either in the morning, before the day started, or in the afternoon to revive herself before dinner. Further, she made it a habit to explore her new surroundings by walking to and from meetings instead of defaulting to a cab.

With a little practice, Casey learned to build routine meal and physical activity habits into her haphazard life. Her mantra became: "A workday is a workday is a workday."

CONCLUSION

BY NOW YOU'VE figured out how to incorporate my daily fixes into your routine. Your job is no longer an excuse for weight gain, and in fact the workday is your greatest asset—the structure it provides facilitates your healthy habits. You are eating well, exercising, and getting enough sleep—at least, more often than not. Hopefully you're also finding time to fit a glass of wine with friends into your busy schedule (and your calorie budget). By proactively planning ahead and using your calendar, you are accountable to yourself and *in control* of your weight and your health—and I mean long-term. And the beauty of it? You feel (and *look*) good.

A lot of people ask me why I became a nutritionist. The truth is, good eating and exercise habits have always been a natural part of my life. When I was growing up, my mother cooked delicious and healthy dinners for our family most nights of the week. Her standard meals usually consisted of fish and stir-fried veggies, always with a side salad with vinaigrette and water for everyone at the table. Her simple, nutritious approach to food and cooking has stuck with me over the years and provides the basis for my "quick-and-easy things to cook" in this book. And my mom wasn't my only healthy influence. My father exercised four nights a week after dinner, around 9:30 p.m., either swimming at the local high school or weight training at the gym. He also spent most Sunday mornings on the track, where he enjoyed running laps (and still does). Growing up, I always assumed it was normal to eat like this and exercise on a regular basis. Creamy salad dressing was for dining out only and soda was reserved for birthday parties. Meals were to be enjoyed and appreciated only after a satisfying workout.

When I went to college, I was privy to disordered eating all around me, and listened to a lot of my girlfriends who were unhappy with themselves and struggling with their weight. Not that I was beyond falling victim to my college lifestyle—certainly, I contended with the rite of passage that is the freshman fifteen. But after eating pizza five nights a week and drinking too much alcohol for a little while, I reverted back to my healthy, childhood habits and lost the weight. My old routine was just more comfortable for me.

When I graduated from college, I felt like I had something to offer my peers in terms of strategies to get healthy. So I applied to a master's program in dietetics. And while grad school and my dietetic internship taught me a lot about the body, disease, and the science of nutrition, I still had the same philosophy about health as I did before all that coursework: Your everyday habits matter most when it comes to a healthy lifestyle.

From the time of this book's inception to today, I have gone through what feels like a million life changes. I moved back and forth between New York City and Cambridge while my husband got an MBA, and even more importantly, I was pregnant for nine months and had my first baby. As a new parent, my son's development and the impact that nutrition has on him are key concerns. I hope to make healthy habits a natural part of his life, so he knows the difference between everyday foods and special-occasion treats to be enjoyed to the fullest.

The Daily Fix was written for my peers and other career women who are ready to get nutrition right once and for all. This is your time to feel energetic, look great, and be confident. *The Daily Fix* supplies a formula for healthy habits, but my hope is that you will be able to ditch calorie counts and food labels once your healthy habits come naturally. At first you will have to make conscious decisions to make better food choices and to exercise more, but my goal for you is that eventually, this lifestyle will become second nature. And by getting it right now, you will be able to instill natural, healthy habits into your children's lives. Remember—obesity is rarely genetic. It is our habits that get passed down from generation to generation that make all the difference.

ENDNOTES

INTRODUCTION

[1] Kane, Leslie. Breaking Bad Habits. *Medical Economics*, March 7, 2007.

CHAPTER 1

[1] Nestle, Marion. *What to Eat: An Aisle-by-Aisle Guide to Savvy Food Choices and Good Eating*. New York: North Point Press, 2006.

[2] Moriyama, Naomi. *Japanese Women Don't Get Old or Fat*. New York: Delacorte Press, 2005.

[3] Wansink, Brian. Environmental factors that increase the food intake and consumption volume of unknowing consumers. *Annual Review of Nutrition* 2004; 455–79.

[4] Kahn BE and Wansink B. The Influence of Assortment Structure on Perceived Variety and Consumption Quantities. *Journal of Consumer Research* 2004; 519–33.

[5] Pucher J and Buehler R. Making Cycling Irresistible: Lessons from the Netherlands, Denmark, and Germany. *Transport Reviews* 2008.

[6] Sallis JF. Environmental and policy interventions to promote physical activity. *American Journal of Preventive Medicine* 1998; 379–97.

[7] Prochaska, James, John Norcross, and Carlo DiClemente. *Changing for Good: A revolutionary six-stage program for overcoming bad habits and moving your life positively forward*. New York: Avon Books, 1995.

CHAPTER 2

[1] Harvard School of Public Health: Fiber, Start Roughing It. http://www.hsph.harvard.edu/nutritionsource/fiber.html. Accessed March 2008.

[2] Pearson, David. Image of a wheat kernel. Created August 2008.

[3] Napoli N et al. Effects of dietary calcium compared with calcium supplements on estrogen metabolism and bone mineral density. *Am J Clin Nutr* 2007; 1428–33.

[4] Guenther PM et al. Most Americans eat much less than recommended amounts of fruits and vegetables. *J Am Diet Assoc* 2006; 1371–79.

[5] Brown WJ et al. Identifying the Energy Gap: Magnitude and Determinants of 5-Year Weight Gain in Midage Women. *Obesity Research* 2005.

CHAPTER 3

[1] Svetkey et al. Comparison of strategies for sustaining weight loss: the weight loss maintenance randomized controlled trial. *JAMA* 2008; 1139–48.

CHAPTER 4

[1] National Organic Program: Revisions to Livestock Standards. *Federal Register*, April 27, 2006.

[2] Raloff, Janet. Hormones: Here's the Beef: environmental concerns reemerge over steroids given to livestock. *Science News*, January 5, 2002.

[3] Balch, Phyllis and James Balch. *Prescription for Nutritional Healing*, Third Edition. New York: Avery 2000.

[4] Lather CM. Role of veterinary medicine in public health: antibiotic use in food animals and humans and the effect on evolution of antibacterial resistance. *J Clin Pharmacol* 2001.

CHAPTER 5

[1] Baker JA et al. Consumption of coffee, but not black tea, is associated with decreased risk of premenopausal breast cancer. *J Nutr* 2006; 166–71.

[2] Inoue M et al. Influence of coffee drinking on subsequent risk of hepatocellular carcinoma: a prospective study in Japan. *J Natl Cancer Inst* 2005; 293–300.

[3] VanDam RM et al. Coffee, caffeine, and risk of type 2 diabetes: a prospective cohort study in younger and middle-aged U.S. women. *Diabetes Care* 2006; 398–403.

[4] Warner, J. Coffee Is No. 1 Source of Antioxidants: Americans Get More Antioxidants from Coffee Than Any Other Food or Beverage. http://www.webmd.com/content/Article/110/109786.htm. Accessed August 2005.

[5] Van Gelder BM et al. Coffee consumption is inversely associated with cognitive decline in elderly European men: the FINE Study. *European Journal of Clinical Nutrition* 2007.

[6] Schwarzschild MA et al. Caffeinated clues and the promise of adenosine A2A antagonists in PD. *Neurology* 2002; 1154–60.

[7] Rodrigues IM and Klein LC. Boiled or filtered coffee? Effects of coffee and caffeine on cholesterol, fibrinogen and C-reactive protein. *Toxicol Rev* 2006; 55–69.

[8] Higdon JV and Frei B. Coffee and health: a review of recent human research. *Crit Rev Food Sci Nutr* 2006; 101–23.

[9] Hallström H et al. Coffee, tea and caffeine consumption in relation to osteoporotic fracture risk in a cohort of Swedish women. *Osteoporos Int* 2006; 1055–64.

[10] McCusker RR et al. Caffeine Content of Decaffeinated Coffee. *Journal of Analytical Toxicology* 2006; 611–13.

[11] Starbucks Coffee Education. www.starbucks.com/ourcoffees/coffee_edu1.a sp?category%5fname=coffee+education. Accessed March 2008.

CHAPTER 6

[1] The National Weight Control Registry. www.nwcr.ws. Accessed March 2008.

[2] Joffe B and Zimmet P. The thrifty genotype in type 2 diabetes. *Endocrine* 1998.

[3] Holt SH et al. The effects of high-carbohydrate vs high-fat breakfasts on feelings of fullness and alertness, and subsequent food intake. *Int J Food Sci Nutr* 1999; 13–28.

[4] Rampersaud GC et al. Breakfast habits, nutritional status, body weight, and academic performance in children and adolescents. *J Am Diet Assoc* 2005; 743–60.

[5] Wolf A et al. A short history of beverages and how our body treats them. *Obes Rev* 2008; 151–64.

[6] Katzen, Mollie and Walter Willet. *Eat Drink and Weigh Less*. New York: Hyperion, 2006.

[7] Gidding et al. Dietary recommendations for children and adolescents: consensus statement from the American Heart Association. *Circulation* 2005.

CHAPTER 7

[1] Forshee, RA et al. A Critical Examination of the Evidence Relating High Fructose Corn Syrup and Weight Gain. *Critical Reviews in Food Science and Nutrition* 2007; 561–82.

CHAPTER 8

[1] Jacobson, MF. Diet & Disease: Time to Act. Available at: http://www. cspinet.org/nah/12_99/cspinews.html. Accessed March 2008.

CHAPTER 9

[1] Drake AJ et al. Bone mineral density and total body bone mineral content in 18- to 22-year-old women. *Bone* 2004.

CHAPTER 10

[1] Dietary Guidelines for Americans 2005—Executive Summary. http://www. health.gov/dietaryguidelines/dga2005/document/html/executivesummary. htm. Accessed March 2008.

[2] Hamid A and Kaur J. Long-term alcohol ingestion alters the folate-binding kinetics in intestinal brush border membrane in experimental alcoholism. *Alcohol* 2007; 441–46.

[3] Rimm EB et al. Review of moderate alcohol consumption and reduced risk of coronary heart disease: is the effect due to beer, wine, or spirits? *BMJ* 1996; 731–36.

[4] Alcohol and the Risk of Breast Cancer. http://envirocancer.cornell.edu/ FactSheet/Diet/fs13.alcohol.cfm. Accessed Mar 2008.

[5] College Alcohol Study: Harvard School of Public Health. http://www.hsph. harvard.edu/cas/. Accessed March 2008.

[6] Wu K et al. Artificially sweetened versus regular mixers increase gastric emptying and alcohol absorption. *AJM* 2006; 802–04.

[7] Trueb RM. Association between smoking and hair loss: another opportunity for health education against smoking? *Dermatology* 2003; 189–91.

[8] Morita A. Tobacco smoke causes premature skin aging. *J Dermatol Sci* 2007; 169–75.

[9] McClernon J et al. The effects of foods, beverages, and other factors on cigarette palatability. *Nicotine & Tobacco Research* 2007; 505–10.

[10] Hasan FM et al. Hypnotherapy as an aid to smoking cessation of hospitalized patients: preliminary results. *Chest Meeting Abstracts* 2007.

CHAPTER 11

[1] Clemens LHE, Slawson DL, and Klesges RC. The Effect of Eating Out on Quality of Diet in Premenopausal Women. *Am Diet Assoc* 1999; 442–44.

[2] Diliberti N et al. Increased Portion Size Leads to Increased Energy Intake in a Restaurant Meal. *Obesity Research* 2004; 562–68.

[3] Ibid.

[4] Christakis NA and Fowler JH. The Spread of Obesity in a Large Social Network over 32 Years. *N Engl J Med* 2007; 370–79.

CHAPTER 12

[1] Larson N et al. Food preparation by young adults is associated with better diet quality. *JADA* 2006; 2001–2007.

[2] Ogle JP and Damhorst ML. Dieting among adolescent girls and their mothers: an interpretative study. *Family and Consumer Research Journal* 2000.

[3] Andersen GS et al. Night eating and weight change in middle-aged men and women. *Int J Obes Relat Metab Disord* 2004; 1338-43.

CHAPTER 13

[1] Patel S. Sleeping Less Linked to Weight Gain. *American Thoracic Society International Conference* 2006.

[2] Spiegel K et al. Brief Communication: Sleep Curtailment in Healthy Young Men is Associated with Decreased Leptin Levels, Elevated Ghrelin Levels, and Increased Hunger and Appetite. *Ann Intern Med* 2004.

[3] 2005 Sleep in America Poll. *National Sleep Foundation* 2005.

[4] Kliff, Sarah. Seven Secrets to a Great Nap: Pining for the perfect siesta? A sleep doc tells us what you need to do for the best midday snooze. *Newsweek*, October 2007.

[5] Parker-Pope, Tara. The Case Against Vitamins: Recent studies show that many vitamins not only don't help. They may actually cause harm. *The Wall Street Journal*, March 20, 2006.

[6] Peters CL et al. An Investigation of Factors That Influence the Consumption of Dietary Supplements. *Health Marketing Quarterly* 2003.

[7] Ansel, Karen. The new message in a bottle: Let thirst be your guide to staying hydrated. www.cookinglight.com/cooking/hl/nutrition/article/0,13803,1697375,00.html. Accessed March 2008.

[8] Peregrin T. C for Yourself: Vitamin C May Slow Skin Wrinkling. *JAMA* 2008; 17.

CHAPTER 14

[1] Blumenthal JA et al. Exercise and pharmacotherapy in the treatment of major depressive disorder. *Psychosomatic Medicine* 2007; 587–96.

[2] Cotman CW et al. Exercise builds brain health: key roles of growth factors cascades and inflammation. *Trends in Neurosciences* 2007; 464–72.

[3] Cheng, Maria. "Thin Fat People?" *The Associated Press*, May 2007.

[4] Levine et al. Interindividual Variation in Posture Allocation: Possible Role in Human Obesity. *Science* 2005.

[5] Hellmich, Nanci. Dieters who exercise may be overeating. http://www.usatoday.com/news/health/2007-10-24-exercise-overeating_N.htm. Accessed March 2008.

CHAPTER 15

[1] Irritable Bowel Syndrome. http://digestive.niddk.nih.gov/ddiseases/pubs/ibs/. Accessed March 2008.

[2] Genital Candidiasis. http://www.cdc.gov/ncidod/dbmd/diseaseinfo/candidiasis_gen_g.htm. Accessed Mar 2008.

[3] Balch, Phyllis and James Balch. *Prescription for Nutritional Healing, Third Edition*. New York: Avery, 2000.

[4] Hassan A and Gordon CM. Polycystic ovary syndrome update in adolescence. *Curr Opin Pediatr* 2007; 389–97.

[5] Balch, Phyllis and James Balch. *Prescription for Nutritional Healing, Third Edition*. New York: Avery, 2000.

[6] Scientists Discover Key to Manipulating Fat. http://explore.georgetown.edu/news/?ID=25475. Accessed March 2008.

[7] Ozier AD et al. Overweight and Obesity Are Associated with Emotion and Stress-Related Eating as Measured by the Eating and Appraisal Due to Emotions and Stress Questionnaire. *JADA* 2008; 49–56.

[8] Shulman KR and Jones GE. The Effectiveness of Massage Therapy Intervention on Reducing Anxiety in the Workplace. *Journal of Applied Behavior Science* 1996.

CHAPTER 16

[1] Rae-Dupree, Janet. Unboxed: Can you become a creature of new habits? *The New York Times*, May 4, 2008.

ACKNOWLEDGMENTS

I'd like to thank my agents Diane Bartoli and Joe Veltre from Artists Literary Group for believing in this first-time author and her book from its inception. Thank you to Susan Berg at Rodale for seeing the potential and then sealing the deal, and to my stellar editor, Julie Will, for her tireless work—you were a godsend. I want to thank *Women's Health* magazine for its endorsement and support, for which I am very grateful.

I also need to thank my amazing husband Birche—you have been my partner in this venture and I could not have done it without you, full stop. I love you. Thanks to my parents and big sister for being naturally healthy and happy people—because of you I was blessed from the start. Thank you thank you thank you to all my HBS friends for supporting me through my stress—I gave birth to this book and my first baby on your watch and could not have gotten through it without your love and kindness. Thanks to my NYU interns Nicole and Samantha—I really appreciate all of your hard work and wish you wellness! Thank you to Leanne—your support for this project has been neverending. Thanks for the recipe help, Amira dear, and the sports nutrition counsel, Carol. And to all my girlfriends and clients who inspired this book, filled out my mini polls, and enthusiastically pushed me forward—you rock! And last but not least, to my dreamy little baby, Miller. Thanks to you, I created Healthy Habit #13: While breastfeeding and writing a book, make sure to eat ice cream every night.

Food Journal

DAY: _____ DATE: _____

TIME	FOOD/DRINK	PORTION	CALORIES	NOTES

Food Journal

DAY: _____ DATE: _____

TIME	FOOD/DRINK	PORTION	CALORIES	NOTES

Food Journal

DAY: _____ DATE: _____

TIME	FOOD/DRINK	PORTION	CALORIES	NOTES

Food Journal

DAY: _____ DATE: _____

TIME	FOOD/DRINK	PORTION	CALORIES	NOTES

FOOD JOURNAL

DAY: _____ DATE: _____

TIME	FOOD/DRINK	PORTION	CALORIES	NOTES

FFQ

FOOD	MON	TUES	WED	THURS	FRI	TOTAL/WEEK
Milk						
Other dairy products						
Fruit						
Vegetables						
Bread						
Rice and other starches						
Cereal/granola bars						
Poultry						
Red meat						
Fish						
Legumes/lentils						
Soy beans/tofu						
Cheese						
Eggs						
Nuts						
Soup						
Olive/canola oil						
Butter						
High-fat snacks						
Low-fat snacks						
Desserts/sweets						
Juice						
Alcohol						
Soda						
Diet soda/drinks						
Coffee						
Tea						

INDEX

Boldfaced page references indicate illustrations. Underscored references indicate boxed text.

C

Caffeine. *See* Coffee
Cage-free food labels, 39
Calcium, 16–17, <u>100</u>, 101–2, <u>102</u>, 154–55, 185
Calendar as nutrition tool, 29–30
Calories
  in alcohol, 110
  burning, amount of, 173
  calculating amount in diet, 21–22, <u>21</u>, <u>22</u>
  counting, 19, 21–22
  defining, 18
  exercise and, <u>165</u>, 172–73
  on food labels, 35
  personal need, 19–21, <u>20</u>, <u>21</u>
  portion sizes and, 21–22
  profile, <u>23</u>
  Quick & Dirty Method, 19
  wasting, avoiding, 93
  weight gain and, <u>16</u>
Candy, 99
Carbohydrates, 13
Carrot soup, 90
Cereal, 65–66, <u>69</u>
Chai tea, <u>57</u>, <u>59</u>
Change, stages of, <u>9–10</u>
Cheese, 79–81, 83, 86
Chewing gum, 182
Chicken, 15, 39, 41, 46, 80, 82, 85, 86, 89, 91, 92, 94, 95, 127, 129, 132, 137, 139, 154, 185
Chinese foods, <u>132–33</u>
Chocolate, dark, 99, <u>105</u>
Cholesterol, 15–16, 110
Cigarettes, 117–19, <u>119</u>
Client dinners, 124–25
Cocktails. *See* Alcohol
Coffee
  caffeine in, 54
  health benefits of, 52–53
  health risks of, 53
  healthy choices, 56–57
  morning habit of, 51
  tea versus, 54–55
  travel mug for, <u>55</u>
Condiments, 87, 93

Constipation, 178–81, <u>179</u>, <u>190</u>
Consumer Lab LLC, 153, <u>153</u>
Cooking, 136–37, <u>139</u>
Corporate resources for exercise, 171
Cottage cheese, 89
Cranberries, 183–84
Cream, 57
Croutons, 83
Crudités, 89
CSA, 40
Culturelle (probiotic), 182

D

Daily Fix. See also Afternoon habits; Evening habits; Morning habits
  design of, xi
  healthy habits of, <u>ix</u>, x
  practicing a habit and, <u>192</u>
  purpose of, 201
  succeeding with, 199–201
  travel and, 191
Daily Value, 36
Dairy foods, 43. *See also specific type*
Dark chocolate, 99, <u>105</u>
Dates, 129–30
Dental health, <u>75</u>
Desserts, 93, 129, 131
Diarrhea, <u>195</u>
Diet. *See* Foods; Nutrition
Dietary fat, 14–16, 83
Diet gimmicks, 6
Diet soda, <u>31</u>, 114
Digestive process, <u>180</u>
Dining out. *See also* Ethnic foods
  appetizers, 123
  dates and, 129–30
  desserts, 129, 131
  girls' night out and, 127–29
  overview, 121
  Plate Method in, 122
  scenarios, common, 129–30
  tips, 121–24
  vegetables and, 129
  weight gain and, <u>122</u>

as side dishes, 140–41
as snacks, 102
steamed, 141
Vegetarian foods, 87
Vinaigrettes, 85
Vitamin C, 159, <u>159</u>
Vitamin D, 155
Vitamin E, 159

W

Walking, 166–68, 171
Water
for afternoon slump, eliminating, 104
alcohol consumption and, alternating with, 114
with dinner, 122
with fiber, for bloating, 161
for hangover relief, 116
hydration and, 157–58
lifestyle habits and, 157–58, <u>157</u>
plane rides and, 193–94
quality of, determining, <u>157</u>
sports drinks versus, 173
thirst and, 157
tips for consuming, 157–58
in treating
constipation, 179–80
irritable bowel syndrome, 181
low libido, 186
premenstrual syndrome, 185
Weight gain
calories and, <u>16</u>
dining out and, <u>122</u>
excuses for, 8–9
polycystic ovary syndrome and, 186
Weight loss
food journal and, <u>25</u>
obstacles to
advertisements for food, 6
environment for exercise, 6–7
overview, 3–4
sugary snack foods, 4
variety of foods, 5–6, <u>5</u>
sleep and, 150
Wendy's (fast food), 95
Wheat, **14**, 37, 161
Whipped cream, avoiding, 57
White wine, 114
Whole grains, 12–14, **14**
Winter squash soup, 90
Work
cereal at, <u>69</u>
client dinners and, 124–25
exercise and, <u>30</u>, 171
fruits at, <u>73</u>
grazing and boredom at, <u>76</u>
lunch meetings at, 92–94
snacks at, <u>103</u>
soups at, <u>94</u>
take-out dinners at, 126–27
Workout schedules, <u>30</u>, 175. *See also* Exercise

Y

Yeast infection, 182–83
Yoga, 118, 144, 165, 169, 170, 171, 175, 189
Yogurt, 89, <u>100</u>

CONVERSION CHART

These equivalents have been slightly rounded to make measuring easier.

VOLUME MEASUREMENTS

U.S.	Imperial	Metric
¼ tsp	–	1 ml
½ tsp	–	2 ml
1 tsp	–	5 ml
1 Tbsp	–	15 ml
2 Tbsp (1 oz)	1 fl oz	30 ml
¼ cup (2 oz)	2 fl oz	60 ml
⅓ cup (3 oz)	3 fl oz	80 ml
½ cup (4 oz)	4 fl oz	120 ml
⅔ cup (5 oz)	5 fl oz	160 ml
¾ cup (6 oz)	6 fl oz	180 ml
1 cup (8 oz)	8 fl oz	240 ml

WEIGHT MEASUREMENTS

U.S.	Metric
1 oz	30 g
2 oz	60 g
4 oz (¼ lb)	115 g
5 oz (⅓ lb)	145 g
6 oz	170 g
7 oz	200 g
8 oz (½ lb)	230 g
10 oz	285 g
12 oz (¾ lb)	340 g
14 oz	400 g
16 oz (1 lb)	455 g
2.2 lb	1 kg

LENGTH MEASUREMENTS

U.S.	Metric
¼"	0.6 cm
½"	1.25 cm
1"	2.5 cm
2"	5 cm
4"	11 cm
6"	15 cm
8"	20 cm
10"	25 cm
12" (1')	30 cm

PAN SIZES

U.S.	Metric
8" cake pan	20 × 4 cm sandwich or cake tin
9" cake pan	23 × 3.5 cm sandwich or cake tin
11" × 7" baking pan	28 × 18 cm baking tin
13" × 9" baking pan	32.5 × 23 cm baking tin
15" × 10" baking pan	38 × 25.5 cm baking tin (Swiss roll tin)
1½ qt baking dish	1.5 liter baking dish
2 qt baking dish	2 liter baking dish
2 qt rectangular baking dish	30 × 19 cm baking dish
9" pie plate	22 × 4 or 23 × 4 cm pie plate
7" or 8" springform pan	18 or 20 cm springform or loose-bottom cake tin
9" × 5" loaf pan	23 × 13 cm or 2 lb narrow loaf tin or pâté tin

TEMPERATURES

Fahrenheit	Centigrade	Gas
140°	60°	–
160°	70°	–
180°	80°	–
225°	105°	¼
250°	120°	½
275°	135°	1
300°	150°	2
325°	160°	3
350°	180°	4
375°	190°	5
400°	200°	6
425°	220°	7
450°	230°	8
475°	245°	9
500°	260°	–

ABOUT THE AUTHOR

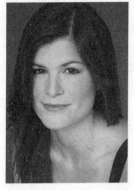

Alexa Levin Fishback was born in Philadelphia. A graduate of the University of Pennsylvania, she went on to complete her nutrition work at New York University and UCSF Medical Center. Currently, Alexa has a private practice focused on weight management and wellness in New York City, where she lives with her husband and son. She practices what she preaches in *The Daily Fix*, cooking, eating well, and working out on a daily basis. This is her first book.

Check out Alexa's Web site at www.alexafishbacknutrition.com